Uterine Diet and Cookbook for Beginner

30+ Quick and Easy Recipes with Delicious Nutrient for Healthy Living (Low-Fibre, Low-Calorie, and Low-Fat)

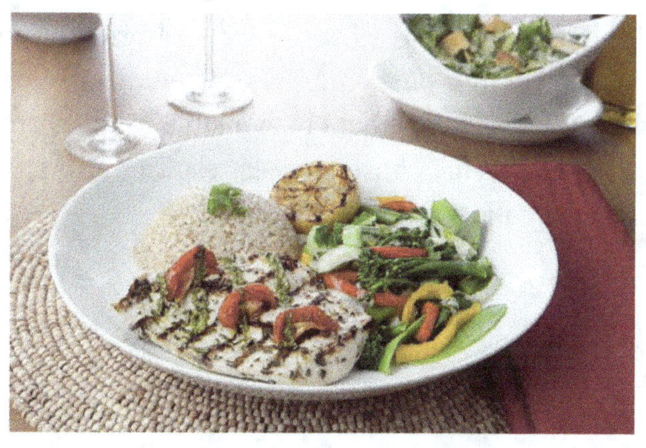

Dr. Mary K. Clubb

Copyright © [2023] by [Dr. Mary K. Clubb]

This book is a work of non-fiction. All of the characters, incidents, and dialogue are drawn from the author's personal experiences, interviews, and research. Any resemblance to actual persons, living or dead, or events is entirely coincidental.

While the author has made every effort to provide accurate and up-to-date information, neither the author nor the publisher can be held responsible for any errors or omissions or for any consequences resulting from the use of this information.

Table of Contents

Introduction

Understanding the Uterus and its Role in Overall Health.

The path to good health often begins on our plates. This idea is particularly applicable to the health of the uterus, a critical organ in a woman's reproductive system. But before we get into the dietary choices that may help you improve your uterine health, let's first explore this extraordinary organ and its significance in your general well-being.

The Uterus: A Powerhouse of Life

The uterus is a pear-shaped muscular organ located inside the pelvis. It plays an integral part in many facets of a woman's life:

- **Menstruation:** During the menstrual cycle, the endometrium, or inner lining of the uterus, thickens in preparation for a possible pregnancy. The lining sheds if pregnancy does not develop, causing a menstrual period.

- **Reproduction:** During pregnancy, the uterus nurtures a fertilized egg as it grows and develops into a baby. The robust muscles contract during labour, enabling the baby to be delivered.

- **Hormonal Regulation:** The uterus also contributes to hormone production, working with the ovaries to maintain a healthy hormonal balance.

The Connection Between Diet and Uterine Health

What we consume dramatically influences the health of all our organs, including the uterus. Here's how a well-balanced diet may help keep your uterus happy and healthy:

- **Chronic inflammation** has been related to a variety of uterine disorders, including fibroids and endometriosis. Anti-inflammatory foods with antioxidants and omega-3 fatty acids may decrease inflammation and improve general health.

- **Hormonal Harmony:** Certain food choices might affect hormone levels. Fibre-rich foods, healthy fats, and specific vitamins and minerals may help balance hormones and lower the risk of uterine problems such as polycystic ovarian syndrome (PCOS).

- **Endometrial Health:** Maintaining a healthy weight and eating meals high in critical nutrients will help to maintain a healthy uterine lining, which is necessary for menstruation and conception.

Adopt a dietary approach to uterine health.

This cookbook will walk you through using food to promote uterine health. We'll look at dishes made with components shown to improve uterine health. Remember, a healthy diet is just one part of the problem. For good uterine health, a comprehensive strategy includes regular exercise, stress management measures, and appropriate Sleep.

Understanding the complicated relationship between your nutrition and uterus will allow you to nurture your body while enjoying your overall health. Let's explore the delectable world of uterine-friendly meals and improve your health one taste at a time!

The Power of Food: Dietary Strategies for Uterine Health Our bodies are inextricably linked, and what we eat significantly influences the health of all organs, including the uterus. By making smart food choices, you may improve your uterine health, encouraging its functioning and lowering your risk of certain illnesses. Let's explore the nutritional practices that might help you maintain a healthy uterus.

1. Fighting Inflammation with Food:

Chronic inflammation has been related to a variety of uterine disorders, including endometriosis and fibroids.

These problems may result in discomfort, irregular periods, and reproductive issues. What is the good news? Anti-inflammatory foods might be your hidden weapon! Fruits and vegetables are high in antioxidants, which help to reduce inflammation. Think about berries, leafy greens, tomatoes, and bell peppers.

- **Omega-3s to the Rescue:** Fatty fish, such as salmon, tuna, and mackerel, contain omega-3 fatty acids, which have been shown to lower inflammation. Aim for a minimum of two servings each week.

- **Spice Up Your Life:** Spices like turmeric, ginger, and cinnamon have powerful anti-inflammatory qualities—experiment with them in your cooking.

2. Promoting Hormonal Harmony:

Hormones play important in releasing the menstrual cycle, ovulation, and mood. Dietary decisions may alter these hormones, affecting uterine health.

- **Fiber is Your Friend:** Fiber regulates blood sugar levels, directly influencing hormone synthesis. Include whole grains, legumes, fruits, and vegetables to ensure a consistent fibre intake.
- Avocados, almonds, and seeds are healthy fats that may help balance hormones. These lipids promote hormone production and control ovulation.

- **Vitamins and Minerals for Support**: Certain vitamins and minerals, such as vitamin E, vitamin D, and magnesium, aid with hormonal equilibrium. Consult your doctor to determine if supplements are essential depending on your specific requirements.

3. Nourishing the endometrium:

The endometrium is the uterine lining, and health is critical for a regular menstrual cycle and conception.

- **Maintain a Healthy Weight:** Being overweight might cause hormone imbalances and influence endometrial health. Aim for a healthy weight by eating a balanced diet and exercising regularly.

- **Nutrient Powerhouse Foods:** Choose foods high in critical nutrients such as folate, iron, and B12. These nutrients promote healthy cell turnover in the endometrium. Leafy green vegetables, lentils, and lean meats are also good sources.

4. Beyond The Plate:

A nutritious diet is an effective tool, but a comprehensive approach is required for maximum uterine health. Consider the following other strategies:

- **Manage Stress:** Stress hormones might alter your menstrual cycle and lead to uterine fibroids. Yoga, meditation, and outdoor time help you manage stress.

- **Move Your Body:** Regular exercise promotes circulation and lowers inflammation, which is helpful to uterine health. Aim for at least 30 minutes of moderate-intensity exercise on most days of the week.

- **Prioritize Sleep:** Sleeping (7-8 hours) is critical for general health, including the uterus. When you are well-rested, your body performs properly, including hormone regulation.

Embrace a Nourishing Journey.

By integrating these nutritional practices and good living behaviours, you may begin a journey to nourish your uterus. Remember that consistency is crucial. This cookbook will be your guide, complete with tasty meals to benefit your uterine health. Explore these recipes and make wise nutritional adjustments to strengthen your body and promote overall well-being, one delicious meal at a time.

Part 1: Establishing the Foundation

Chapter One: Essential Nutrients for Uterine Health

1.1 Anti-inflammatory Powerhouses.

Chronic inflammation is a hidden cause of many health problems, and the uterus is no different. It has been connected to disorders such as endometriosis, fibroids, and irregular periods. But don't worry, Mother Nature has plenty of anti-inflammatory powerhouses that can help you promote uterine wellness! Let's look at some crucial actors and how they may help your well-being:

1. Antioxidant All-Stars:

These bright fruits and vegetables are high in antioxidant chemicals, which fight inflammation by neutralizing damaging free radicals in the body. Here are several champions to include on your plate:

- **Berry Bonanza:** Berries, including blueberries, strawberries, raspberries, and cherries, are high in antioxidants like anthocyanin. These powerful ingredients may help decrease inflammation, including the uterus.

- **Leafy Green Giants:** Dark leafy greens like kale, spinach, and collard greens are high in antioxidants such as vitamins A, C, and E. These essential nutrients reduce inflammation and promote overall wellness.

- **Cruciferous Crusaders:** The cruciferous family includes vegetables like broccoli, cauliflower, Brussels sprouts, and cabbage. They are high in sulforaphane, an anti-inflammatory substance that may be especially useful for uterine health.

- **Tomatoes & Lycopene:** This brilliant red fruit (yes, it is a fruit!) contains lycopene, a powerful antioxidant with anti-inflammatory qualities. Cooked tomatoes are an even higher source of lycopene, so eat them in tomato sauce, salsa, or roast!

2. Omega 3 Odyssey:

Omega-3 fatty acids are necessary lipids with significant anti-inflammatory properties. Here's how adding them to your diet may help your uterus:

- **Fatty Fish Feast:** Salmon, tuna, mackerel, sardines, and herring are high in omega-3 fatty acids, namely EPA and DHA. Consume at least two servings of these fish weekly to gain the anti-inflammatory effects.

- **Plant-Based Options:** Walnuts, flaxseeds, and chia seeds are high in alpha-linolenic acid (ALA), an omega-3 fatty acid that vegetarians and vegans may benefit from. Your body can convert ALA to EPA and DHA, although less effectively than fish.

3. *Spice up your life with anti-inflammatory power.*

Certain spices not only add taste to your food, but they also have potent anti-inflammatory qualities. Here are a few spices to include in your anti-inflammatory arsenal:

- **Turmeric Triumph:** Turmeric, the golden spice, contains curcumin, a potent anti-inflammatory agent. Combine turmeric with black pepper to increase curcumin absorption.

- **Ginger's Soothing Power:** For millennia, ginger has been utilized for therapeutic purposes. Its anti-inflammatory properties may benefit uterine health and aid with menstrual cramps.

- **Cinnamon's Sweet Relief:** Aside from its pleasant scent, cinnamon has anti-inflammatory qualities that may help decrease inflammation throughout the body.

Making the Most of Anti-inflammatory Powerhouses.

Variety is Important: Don't restrict yourself to a single anti-inflammatory powerhouse. Explore various fruits, vegetables, seafood, and spices to understand nutrients with anti-inflammatory properties.

Fruits and vegetables, whether fresh or frozen, may be good providers of antioxidants. Frozen alternatives are often flash-frozen at peak ripeness, retaining their nutritional value.

Cooking processes Matter: Certain cooking processes may increase the availability of anti-inflammatory chemicals. For example, steaming or briefly stir-frying veggies helps to preserve their antioxidant content.

Including these anti-inflammatory superfoods in your diet may build a natural barrier against inflammation and maintain a healthy uterus. Remember that consistency is crucial! The more you adopt these nutritional recommendations, the more you'll improve your general health. This cookbook will give you tasty dishes, including these anti-inflammatory superstars, making feeding your body more straightforward and supporting uterine health.

1.2 Balance Hormones Naturally

The human body is a beautiful orchestra, with hormones conducting a complicated symphony of operations. When these hormones work in tandem, a sensation of well-being spreads throughout. However, for many women, hormone imbalances may interrupt this symphony, resulting in a slew of symptoms that can harm the uterus. Do not worry, maestro! Understanding the power of food and adopting natural solutions may help you become the conductor of your hormonal harmony, resulting in a healthy and vibrant uterus.

The Delicate Dance of Hormones

Estrogen, progesterone, and a few more hormones collaborate in a complex ballet to control your menstrual cycle, ovulation, and mood. When this dance gets out of sync, it may result in irregular periods, mood swings, and even reproductive problems. Conditions such as polycystic ovarian syndrome (PCOS) may further alter hormonal balance, affecting uterine health.

Nature's Tuning Fork: Foods for Hormone Balance

Particular food choices may serve like a tuning fork, gently coaxing your hormones back into balance. Here are some crucial components to include in your everyday repertoire:

Fiber Fiesta: Fiber works like a gentle sweeper, removing extra hormones from your system. Fibre-rich foods include whole grains, legumes, fruits, and vegetables.

The good Fat Symphony: Don't avoid good fats like avocado, almonds, and seeds. These lipids are required for hormone synthesis and to control ovulation. Consider them the instruments needed for the hormonal orchestra to play.

The Vitamin and Mineral Chorus: Vitamins E, D, and magnesium are essential in the hormonal symphony. Foods high in these vital elements include leafy green vegetables, lentils, and lean meats. If necessary, visit a doctor to establish if supplements are required to support your specific hormonal demands.

Beyond the Plate: Practices for Hormonal Harmony

A nutritious diet is an effective conductor, but a comprehensive strategy is required for a harmonious hormonal symphony. Consider the following extra practices:

Manage the Stressful Crescendo: Stress hormones may cause hormonal imbalance. Yoga, meditation, and time in nature help you manage stress and restore balance to your hormones.

Move Your Body for a Balanced Rhythm: Regular exercise increases circulation and decreases inflammation, which are both helpful to hormonal health. Aim for 30 minutes of moderate-intensity exercise most days of the week to keep your body moving in a healthy rhythm.

Prioritize Sleep, the Sweet Lullaby: Getting enough Sleep (7-8 hours) helps your body reset and optimize all of its activities, including hormonal balance. When well-rested, the hormonal symphony can be performed quickly and efficiently.

Embracing the Balanced Journey:

By integrating these nutritional and lifestyle practices, you may take control of your hormonal symphony and promote a healthy and happy uterus. Remember that consistency is crucial. This cookbook will guide you with tasty meals to help with hormonal balance. As you experiment with these recipes and make wise food choices, you'll balance your hormones and create a symphony of well-being, one delicious mouthful at a time.

1.3 Strengthening the Uterine Lining

The endometrium, or uterine lining, is essential for menstruation and fertilization. It's like a fertile environment where a fertilized egg may implant and develop into a healthy kid. However, a thin or diseased endometrium may impede this process. But don't worry!

Particular dietary practices may help to nourish and grow your endometrium, laying the groundwork for a healthy reproductive system.

Understanding the endometrium:

The endometrium goes through a monthly cycle, thickening in preparation for a possible pregnancy and shedding during menstruation. During the mid-luteal phase (the time after ovulation), a healthy endometrium measures around 7-10 millimeters thick. Weight, age, and hormone imbalances all impact endometrial thickness and health.

Dietary strategies for a strong endometrium:

Let's examine some dietary choices that help maintain a healthy and robust endometrium.

- **Maintaining a Healthy Weight:** Being overweight or obese may cause hormone imbalances and harm endometrial health. Aim for a healthy weight by eating a balanced diet and exercising regularly.

- **Fueling with Folate:** Folate, a B vitamin, is essential for cell development and repair, especially in the endometrium. Leafy green vegetables, lentils, and fortified grains are rich in folate.

- **Iron for a Strong Foundation:** Iron insufficiency may cause a thin endometrium and irregular periods. Lean meats, fish, beans, and iron-fortified meals such as cereals may help keep iron levels stable.

- **Vitamin B12 for Optimal Functioning:** Vitamin B12 is a critical ingredient for cell development and division, which is required for a healthy endometrium. Salmon, eggs, and fortified cereals are excellent sources of Vitamin B12.

Beyond the Plate: Practices for Endometrial Health.

While a good diet is crucial, the following lifestyle activities may further promote a robust endometrium:

- **Limit Refined Carbs:** Refined carbs may raise blood sugar levels, alter hormone synthesis, and affect the endometrium. Choose whole grains instead, which give lasting energy and are high in healthy elements.

- Reduce your consumption of processed foods and trans fats since they may cause inflammation and impact general health, including the endometrium. For the best nourishment, eat entire, unprocessed foods.

Chapter 2: Stocking your pantry: uterine-friendly staples

2.1 Whole grains and legumes

Two nutritional measures for a healthy uterus stand out: whole grains and legumes. These diverse components, high in critical nutrients and with several health advantages, deserve to be prominent in your uterine-friendly diet. Let's examine why whole grains and legumes are great for uterine health and how to integrate them into your diet.

Whole grains are nature's nutritional powerhouse.

Unlike refined grains, which have been stripped of their bran and germ, whole grains maintain all of the kernel's components: bran, germ, and endosperm. This results in a variety of nutrients, including:

- **Fibre:** Whole grains are high in fibre, essential for digestive health and hormone control. Fibre makes you feel full, regulates blood sugar levels, and aids in absorbing excess hormones.

- **B vitamins** are essential in early generation, cell development, and nervous system function. Whole grains are high in B vitamins necessary for maintaining a healthy hormonal balance.

- **Minerals:** Whole grains provide vital minerals such as magnesium, iron, and zinc, all of which promote general health and may indirectly benefit uterine health.

Legume Love: A Nutritional Treasure Trove.

Legumes, often known as pulses, include various foods such as beans, lentils, chickpeas, and peas. Legumes, like whole grains, have several health advantages for the uterus, including:

- **Plant-Based Protein Powerhouse:** Legumes are an excellent source of plant-based protein, which is required for tissue growth and repair. Protein also regulates hormones and promotes a healthy metabolism.

- **Fibre Fiesta:** Legumes, like whole grains, are high in fibre, which promotes digestive health and helps regulate hormones.

- **Iron Rich:** Iron deficiency may cause irregular periods and exhaustion. Legumes are an excellent source of iron, especially for women with excessive menstrual flow.

- **Folate Friend:** This critical B vitamin promotes cell growth and development, which helps to maintain a healthy endometrium. Legumes are high in folate, which supports reproductive health.

Deliciously Diverse: How to Enjoy Whole Grains and Legumes.

Whole grains and legumes are appealing due to their flexibility. Here's how you can add them to your diet for a uterine-friendly feast:

- **Breakfast Bonanza:** Start the day with a breakfast of fibre-rich whole-grain oats or quinoa. Legumes may also be a morning staple; try a lentil stew or a chickpea scramble.

- Salads with healthy grains and lentils provide a light and healthful lunch choice. Tossing whole-wheat spaghetti with lentils and veggies makes for a filling and nutritious supper.

- **Meal Delights:** Get creative with your meal! Fajitas made with whole-grain tortillas, black beans, and veggies are excellent. Warm and comforting alternatives include hearty lentil soup and chickpea curry.

This cookbook will include a range of dishes that use healthy grains and legumes, making it simple to integrate these superfoods into your uterine-friendly diet.

Remember that even little modifications may have a significant effect. Gradually including whole grains and legumes into your diet will feed your body and promote uterine health while enjoying tremendous and fulfilling cuisine.

2.2 Fruit and Vegetables

Mother Nature gives a brilliant variety of fruits and vegetables, and when it comes to uterine health, these beautiful jewels prove to be effective partners. Fruits and vegetables are high in essential nutrients, antioxidants, and fibre, which are vital in maintaining a healthy and happy uterus. Let's look further into their precise advantages and find beautiful ways to include them in your diet.

A Rainbow of Benefits:

Fruits and vegetables have various nutrients that contribute to general health and, indirectly, uterine well-being. Here are some significant highlights:

- **Antioxidant Powerhouses:** Fruits and vegetables are loaded with antioxidants that fight free radicals, which cause inflammation and chronic illnesses. The antioxidants' anti-inflammatory qualities are beneficial to a healthy uterus.

- **Fiber Fiesta:** Fiber helps you feel full, regulates blood sugar levels, and assists in hormone clearance. This may be especially useful for controlling menstruation discomfort and supporting hormonal balance.

Fruits and vegetables include critical vitamins and minerals such as C, E, folate, iron, and magnesium. These nutrients are essential for general health and indirectly contribute to a healthy reproductive system.

Specific Powerhouses of Uterine Health:

While all fruits and vegetables have advantages, several stand out for their unique contributions to uterine health:

Berries: These tasty berries (blueberries, raspberries, strawberries) are high in antioxidants and may help decrease inflammation, which has been related to illnesses such as endometriosis.

Leafy Greens: Dark leafy greens, including kale, spinach, and collard greens, are high in folate, which is necessary for cell growth and development, particularly in the endometrium.

Cruciferous vegetables include broccoli, cauliflower, Brussels sprouts, and cabbage, which contain substances that may help control estrogen levels, possibly lowering the risk of uterine fibroids.

Tomatoes: This bright fruit (yes, a food!) contains lycopene, an antioxidant that may aid heart and uterine health.

Beyond the Plate: Maximizing Benefits:

To maximize the advantages of fruits and vegetables:

Variety is essential: Do not restrict yourself to a few favourites. To receive a more diversified spectrum of nutrients, try a variety of fruits and vegetables.

Fruits and vegetables, whether fresh or frozen, may be good vitamin sources. Frozen alternatives are often flash-frozen at peak ripeness, retaining their nutritional value.

Cooking procedures Matter: Certain cooking procedures may increase the availability of specific nutrients. Steaming or briefly stir-frying veggies preserves their antioxidant content.

A Culinary Adventure: Delicious Ways to Enjoy Fruits and Vegetables.

Fruits and vegetables are very adaptable, allowing for many culinary combinations. Here are some suggestions for including them in your uterine-friendly diet.

- **Breakfast Bliss:** Begin the day with a smoothie with berries, spinach, and banana. Pair fresh fruit slices with yoghurt or porridge.

- **Lunchtime Highlights:** Salads are an excellent way to include a range of fruits and vegetables.

Grill veggies for a smokey taste, or mix chopped fruits into your favourite salad.

- **Dinner Delights:** Serve a colourful mix of veggies as a side. Stuff bell peppers with quinoa and chopped veggies for a robust and filling supper.

2.3 Healthy Fats and Proteins

Two critical characteristics on our path to improving uterine health characteristics choices: healthy fats and protein. These powerhouses each perform a unique but critical function in laying the groundwork for a healthy reproductive system. Let's look further into their precise advantages and find beautiful ways to include them in your diet.

Healthy Fats: Fuel for Your Body and Beyond:

Contrary to common opinion, not all fats are created equally. Healthy fats are essential for many body processes, including:

- **Hormone synthesis:** Certain healthy fats are precursors for hormone synthesis, promoting hormonal equilibrium. This is especially crucial for managing the menstrual cycle and ovulation.

- **Nutrient Absorption:** Healthy fats absorb fat-soluble vitamins such as A, D, E, and K. These vitamins are essential for general health and indirectly promote uterine health.

- **Cellular Health:** Healthy lipids are necessary components of cell membranes, which promote healthy cell activity throughout the body, including the uterus.

Selecting the Suitable Fats for Uterine Health:

To promote uterine health, consider these healthy fat sources:

- **Monounsaturated fats** are found in avocados, olive oil, nuts (almonds, cashews), and seeds (flaxseeds, chia seeds), providing several health advantages.

- **Polyunsaturated Fats:** Essential polyunsaturated fats include omega-3 and omega-6. Fatty fish (such as salmon, tuna, and sardines) are high in omega-3s, essential for reducing inflammation. Plant-based sources of omega-3s include walnuts, flaxseeds, and chia seeds.

Protein: The Building Blocks of a Healthy Uterus.

Protein is another essential ingredient for a healthy reproductive system. Here's why.

- Protein is used to construct and repair tissues throughout the body, including the endometrium. A healthy endometrium is essential for implantation during pregnancy.

- **Hormone Regulation:** Certain proteins serve as precursors for hormone synthesis, helping to maintain a balanced hormonal environment.

- **Energy Production:** While protein is not the primary energy source, it may be utilized as fuel, particularly during calorie restriction.

Choose Protein Sources for Uterine Health:

Prioritize these protein sources to help your uterine health.

- **Lean Protein Sources:** Lean meats, poultry, and fish have high-quality protein with less saturated fat.

- **Plant-Based Protein Powerhouses:** Legumes (beans, lentils), tofu, tempeh, and almonds are high-quality plant-based protein sources ideal for vegetarians and vegans.

- **Eggs:** Eggs are a flexible and economical protein source containing all necessary amino acids.

Creating A Balanced Plate: Combining Healthy Fats and Protein

The secret is balancing healthy fats and protein to produce balanced and enjoyable meals. Here are a few tips:

- **Pair Protein with Healthy Fats:** Include a source of healthy fat in each meal that contains protein. For example, try grilled chicken with avocado slices or baked salmon with roasted veggies drizzled with olive oil.

- **Snack Smart:** To make enjoyable snacks, combine protein and healthy fats. Serve apple slices with almond butter, Greek yoghurt with berries and chia seeds, or a handful of mixed nuts.

A Culinary Adventure: Delicious Ways to Eat Healthy Fats and Protein

Healthy fats and protein may be blended into a wide range of cuisines, making healthy and pleasurable meals. Here are a few ideas:

- **Breakfast Delights:** Delicious and protein-rich alternatives include scrambled eggs with veggies and avocado slices, Greek yoghurt with berries and almonds, and a protein smoothie with nut butter and spinach.

- **Lunchtime Powerhouses:** Protein-packed lunch options include salads with grilled chicken or tofu, lentil soup with a whole-wheat roll, and a veggie burger on a whole-wheat bun, all of which may be coupled with a healthy fat source like avocado or olive oil dressing.

- **Dinnertime Duos:** For a substantial meal, try baked salmon with roasted veggies, a stir-fry with lean protein and mixed vegetables drizzled with sesame oil, or lentil stew with a dollop of Greek yoghurt.

Part 2: Delicious Meals for Every Day

Chapter 3: Breakfast Delights.

3.1 High Fiber Porridge with Berries and Nuts

High-fiber porridge with berries and nuts

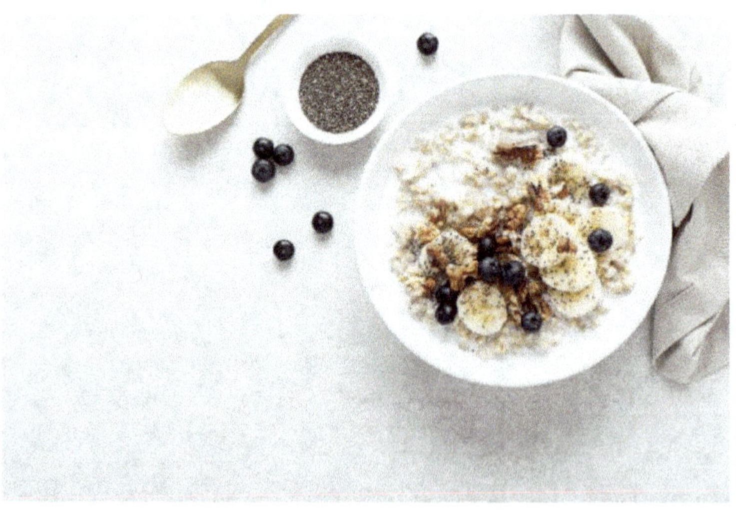

This meal is a tasty and healthful way to begin the day. It's high in fibre, antioxidants, and protein, making it great for improving uterine health.

Ingredients:

- ½ cup rolled oats, old-fashioned or quick.
- One cup of unsweetened plant-based milk (almond, soy, or oat).
- ¼ cup water.
- One tablespoon of ground flaxseed (optional)
- ¼ cup mixed berries, fresh or frozen.
- ¼ cup chopped nuts (almonds, walnuts, and pecans).
- One tablespoon of chia seeds (optional).
- Half a teaspoon of crushed cinnamon
- A pinch of salt is optional.
- Sweeten to taste (maple syrup, honey, agave nectar, etc.).

Instructions:

1. Mix the rolled oats, plant-based milk, water, flaxseed (if using), and cinnamon in a saucepan. Bring to a boil over medium heat.

2. Reduce the heat to low and simmer for 5-7 minutes until the oats are cooked and the porridge achieves the desired consistency. If the porridge gets too thick, add more milk or water.

3. While the oatmeal is cooking, prepare your toppings. If not previously chopped, chop the nuts and defrost any frozen berries.

4. After cooking, remove the porridge from the heat and whisk in the mixed berries and chia seeds (if using).

5. Place the porridge in a bowl and garnish with chopped nuts, a drizzle of your choice sweetener (optional), and a teaspoon of salt.

Tips:

- To make a creamier porridge, use more milk and less water.
- If you don't have ground flaxseed, you may grind whole flaxseeds in a spice or coffee grinder before putting them in the kettle.
- You may use various kinds of nuts and berries depending on your preferences.
- To make this dish vegan, use plant-based milk and skip honey as a sweetener.

This porridge may be refrigerated in an airtight container for up to three days. Reheat gently in a pot or microwave before serving.

Berry Chia Pudding With Toasted Nuts

This overnight oats version is another excellent high-fibre breakfast choice. It's ideal for meal planning since it can be made the night before.

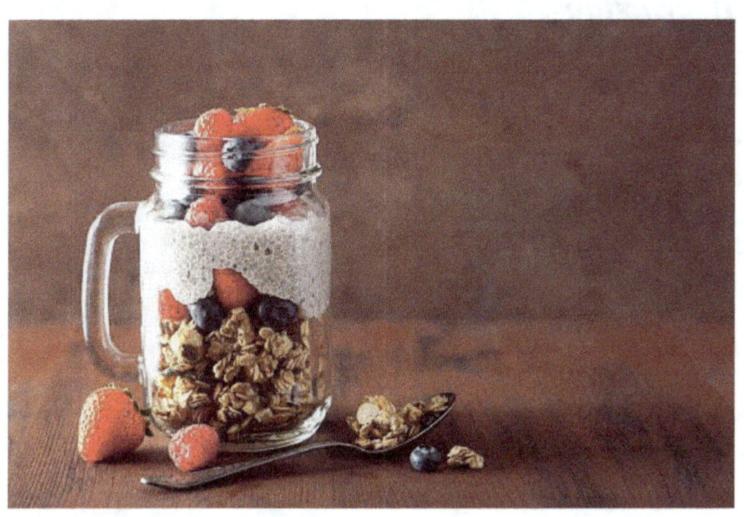

Ingredients:

- ½ cup rolled oats, old-fashioned or quick.
- ½ cup of unsweetened plant-based milk (e.g., almond, soy, or oat).
- ¼ cup chia seeds.
- ¼ cup mixed berries, fresh or frozen.
- ¼ cup chopped nuts (almonds, walnuts, and pecans).
- One tablespoon of maple syrup (or another sweetener)
- ½ teaspoon of vanilla extract (optional)
- A pinch of ground cinnamon.

Instructions:

1. Mix the rolled oats, plant-based milk, chia seeds, maple syrup, vanilla extract (if using), and cinnamon in a jar or container with a cover. Stir well to combine.

2. Fold in the mixed berries.

3. Place the cover on the jar and refrigerate overnight or for at least 6 hours.

4. In the morning, remix the chia pudding. Top with chopped nuts, and enjoy!

Tips:

- Spread the nuts on a baking sheet and toast in a preheated oven at 350°F (175°C) for 5-7 minutes until aromatic and golden brown. Pay special attention to prevent burning.
- To suit your tastes, you may make this recipe with various kinds of milk, berries, nuts, and sweeteners.

This chia pudding may be refrigerated in an airtight container for up to three days.
Enjoy these nutritious and tasty high-fibre porridge dishes as part of your uterine-healthy diet!

3.2 Scrambled eggs with spinach and feta cheese.

This dish is a fast, protein-packed, and tasty addition to any dinner. It's high in nutrients that may help maintain a healthy uterus, making it an ideal complement to your uterine-friendly diet.

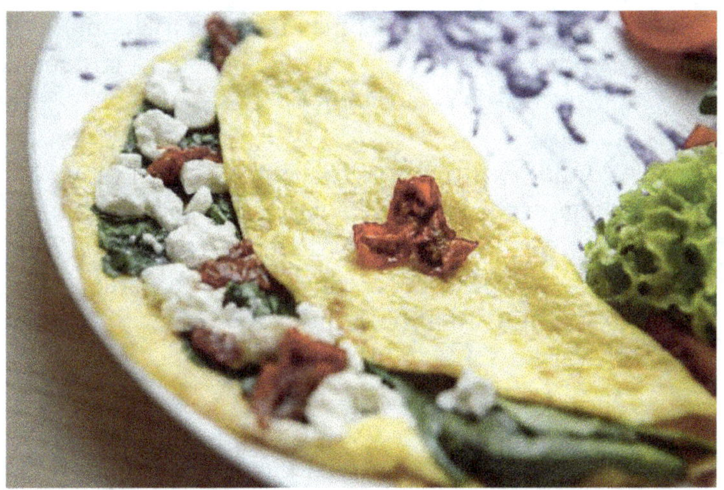

Ingredients:

- Three huge eggs.
- One tablespoon of unsalted butter.
- One cup of baby spinach, coarsely chopped.
- ¼ cup crumbled feta cheese.
- ¼ teaspoon of dried oregano (optional)
- Add salt and freshly cracked black pepper to taste.

Instructions:

1. Crack the eggs into a mixing dish and whisk until thoroughly mixed—season with salt and pepper.

2. Heat the butter in a nonstick pan over medium heat. Once the butter has melted, swirl it to coat the pan.

3. Cook the chopped spinach in the pan, moving periodically, until wilted and softened, approximately 1-2 minutes.

4. Add the whisked eggs to the pan with the spinach. Using a rubber spatula, carefully push the cooked egg from the pan's borders toward the middle, enabling the uncooked egg to fill the area. Continue to boil and whisk gently until the eggs are almost set but still a little moist.

5. Remove the skillet from the heat and scatter the feta cheese over the eggs. Gently incorporate the cheese into the eggs, allowing it to melt slightly from the remaining heat.

6. Season with salt and pepper to taste, then garnish with dried oregano (if using).

7. Serve immediately with whole wheat bread or a side salad for a complete and balanced dinner.

Tips:

- Mix in a splash of milk or water (approximately one tablespoon) to make creamier scrambled eggs before frying them.
- If you don't have fresh spinach, you may use frozen spinach. Thaw the spinach well and wring off any extra liquid before adding it to the pan.
- Depending on your preferences, crumbled goat or ricotta cheese may be used instead of feta cheese.
- To make this meal vegetarian, leave out the feta cheese. The meal will remain protein-rich and flavorful.
- A sprinkle of red pepper flakes may be added to the whisked eggs for a spicy kick.

Variations:

- **Sun-dried Tomato and Basil:** For a Mediterranean flavour, combine chopped sun-dried tomatoes and a sprinkling of dried basil in the skillet with the spinach.
- Sauté cubed ham and chopped onion in a skillet before adding the spinach. Continue with the recipe as directed.
- **Mushrooms and Herbs:** Saute sliced mushrooms in a skillet before adding spinach—season with a pinch of rosemary or dried thyme.

Enjoy this protein-rich and tasty Scrambled Eggs with Spinach & Feta Cheese dish as part of a uterine-healthy diet!

3.3 Green Power Smoothie with Fruits and Seeds

Smoothies are a delightful and handy way to get plenty of nutrients into your diet. These vivid concoctions, which include greens, fruits, and seeds, are great for uterine health because they provide critical nutrients and promote a balanced hormone balance. Let's look at three different smoothie recipes with distinct taste and health advantages.

Tropical Green Goddess

This refreshing smoothie is a delicious combination of tropical fruits, leafy greens, and healthy fats that will satisfy your taste buds while nourishing your body.

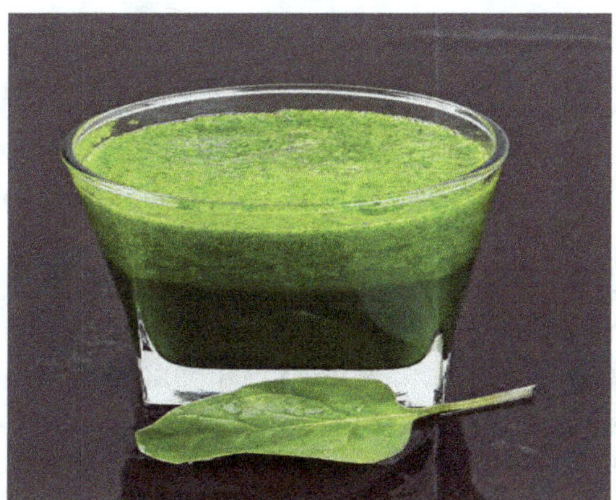

Ingredients:

- 1 cup of unsweetened plant-based milk (almond, coconut, etc.)
- ½ cup of frozen mango chunks.
- ¼ cup chopped pineapple.
- One handful (about one cup) of fresh spinach
- One tablespoon of ground flaxseed.
- ½ banana, fresh or frozen.
- One tablespoon of nut butter (almond, cashew, etc.)
- ½ teaspoon of ground ginger (optional)
- A pinch of ground turmeric (optional).

Instructions:

1. Blend all of the ingredients until smooth and creamy. If the smoothie is too thick, add a splash

of plant-based milk to get the appropriate consistency.

2. Pour in a glass and enjoy!

Benefits: This smoothie has a wealth of nutrients. Mango and pineapple supply vitamin C and antioxidants, while spinach contains folate and iron. Flaxseed and nut butter provide healthful fats and fibre, while ginger and turmeric provide anti-inflammatory benefits.

Berrylicious Blast

This antioxidant-rich smoothie is loaded with berries and greens, producing delicious flavour and improving overall health.

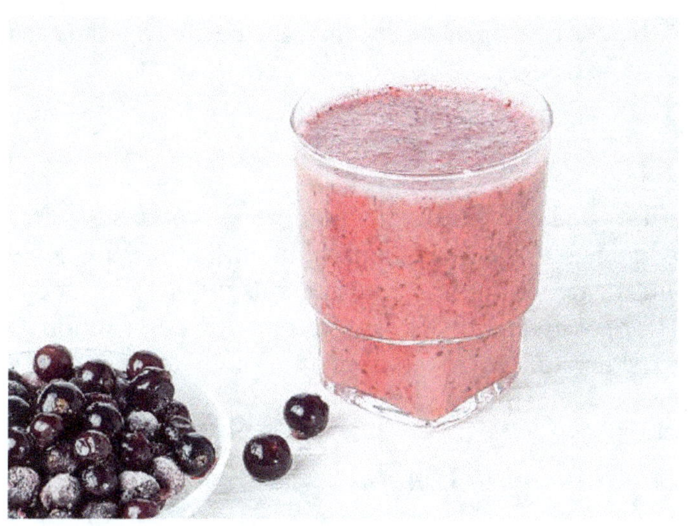

Ingredients:

- 1 cup water.
- One cup of frozen mixed berries (blueberries, raspberries, and strawberries).
- ½ cup of chopped baby kale.
- ½ banana, fresh or frozen.
- One tablespoon of chia seeds.
- One scoop of vanilla protein powder (optional).
- A handful of ice cubes (optional)

Instructions:

1. Blend all of the ingredients until smooth and creamy. If the smoothie is overly thick, add extra

water or a splash of plant-based milk to adjust the consistency.

2. Pour in a glass and enjoy!

Benefits: This bright smoothie contains berry antioxidants, which may help fight inflammation. Kale contains critical vitamins and minerals, whilst chia seeds give fibre and healthy fats. Protein powder (optional) provides an additional source of protein to promote a healthy reproductive system.

Green Glow with Matcha

This innovative smoothie combines greens, bananas, and matcha powder to create a creamy and refreshing beverage.

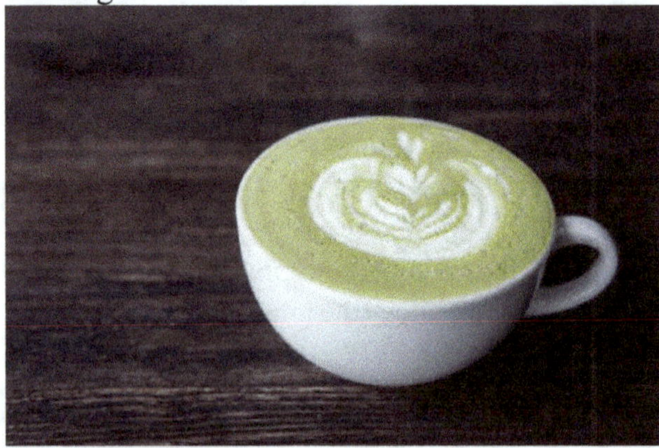

Ingredients:

- One cup of unsweetened almond milk.

- One cup of fresh spinach or romaine lettuce.
- ½ banana, fresh or frozen.
- One spoonful of plain Greek yoghurt.
- One teaspoon of matcha powder.
- ½ teaspoon of honey or maple syrup (optional)

Instructions:

1. Blend all of the ingredients until smooth and creamy. If the smoothie is too thick, add a splash of almond milk to get the required consistency.
2. Pour in a glass and enjoy!

Benefits: This stimulating smoothie contains greens, which provide critical vitamins and minerals. Banana provides natural sweetness and potassium, while Greek yoghurt contains protein and bacteria. Matcha powder has a distinct taste and provides a modest energy boost, while honey or maple syrup (optional) adds a hint of sweetness.

These are just a handful of the many choices for making power smoothies for uterine health. Feel free to experiment with various fruits, veggies, and seeds. Use milk substitutes to find your preferred taste combinations. Remember that consistency is crucial! Including these vivid smoothies in your diet will supply your body with the nutrients it needs for a healthy uterus while enjoying tasty and refreshing drinks.

Chapter 4: Vibrant Salads and Bowls

4.1 Quinoa salad with roasted vegetables and tahini dressing.

This colourful quinoa salad is a symphony of textures and tastes, packed with roasted veggies and a creamy tahini dressing. It's a substantial and fulfilling meal that may be served as a light lunch, side dish, or vegetarian main course. This meal celebrates fresh, seasonal food while providing a well-balanced supply of protein, fibre, healthy fats, and critical vitamins for uterine health.

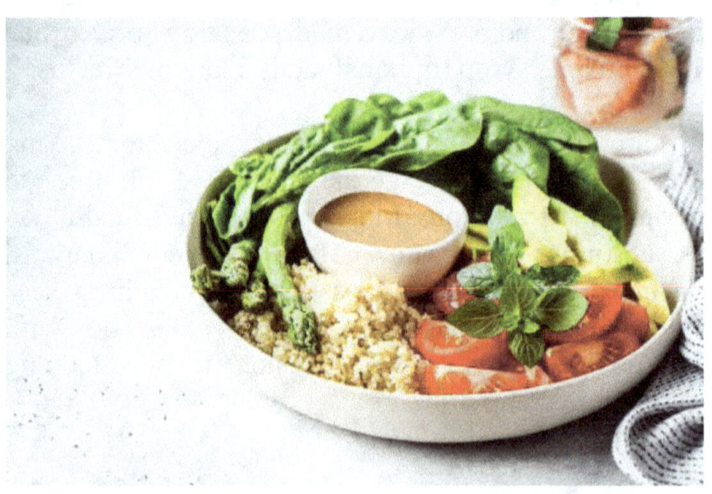

Ingredients:

For the quinoa:

- 1 cup of quinoa, rinsed
- One ¾ cup veggie broth.
- ½ teaspoon salt.

For the roasted vegetables:

- One medium red bell pepper, chopped.
- One medium yellow bell pepper, chopped.
- One medium zucchini, chopped.
- One medium red onion, chopped.
- One tablespoon of olive oil.
- ½ teaspoon dried oregano.
- ¼ teaspoon salt
- ¼ teaspoon black pepper.

For Tahini Dressing:

- ¼ cup tahini paste
- Two teaspoons of lemon juice.
- Two tablespoons olive oil.
- Two garlic cloves, minced
- Two tablespoons water (add more if necessary)
- ¼ teaspoon ground cumin
- Pinch of salt.

For the salad:

- ½ cup crumbled feta cheese (optional).
- ¼ cup chopped fresh parsley.
- ¼ cup chopped fresh mint.

Instructions:

Cook the Quinoa:
1. Mix the rinsed quinoa, vegetable broth, and salt in a medium saucepan.
2. Bring to a boil over medium heat.
3. Reduce the heat, cover the pan, and cook for 15-20 minutes or until the quinoa is fully cooked and fluffy.
4. Remove from heat and let to fluff with a fork for 5 minutes.
5. Set aside to cool somewhat.

Preheat the oven to 400:
1. Preheat) to roast the vegetables.
2. On a baking sheet with parchment paper.
3. Oss the chopped red and yellow bell peppers, zucchini, and red onion with olive oil, oregano, salt, and pepper.
4. Read the veggies on the prepared baking sheet and roast for 20-25 minutes or until soft and lightly browned.

- Remove from the oven and let it cool slightly.

- **Make the Tahini Dressing**: In a small mixing bowl, combine tahini paste, lemon juice, olive oil, chopped garlic, cumin, and salt. Whisk in the water one tablespoon until the dressing achieves the required consistency (creamy yet pourable).
- **Prepare the Salad:** In a large mixing bowl, add the cooled quinoa, roasted veggies, crumbled feta cheese (if using), and chopped parsley and mint. Pour the tahini dressing over the salad and gently toss to cover all components evenly.

- Serve, and enjoy! Plate your vivid quinoa salad and serve at room temperature or slightly cold.

Tips:

- To save time, use precooked quinoa. However, cleaning and boiling your quinoa gives you more control over texture and taste.
- Feel free to alter the veggies to your liking. Other excellent choices are broccoli florets, Brussels sprouts, and sliced asparagus.
- If you don't have fresh herbs, use one teaspoon of dried parsley or mint for the chopped fresh ones.
- Refrigerate leftovers in an airtight jar for up to three days.

This quinoa salad with roasted carrots and tahini dressing is a delicious and nutritious addition to your uterine-healthy eating plan. It's a gorgeous and savoury meal that will fuel your body while pleasing your taste senses!

4.2 Lentil Soup With Kale And Whole Wheat Bread

With this hearty lentil soup dish, you'll feel like you're being hugged. This dinner is a symphony of textures and tastes, with protein-rich lentils, iron-fortified kale, and all the deliciousness of handmade whole wheat bread. It is not only delicious, but it also provides your body with critical nutrients that support a healthy uterus. Let's look at how to make this healthy cuisine ideal for a lovely night in or a delicious lunch party.

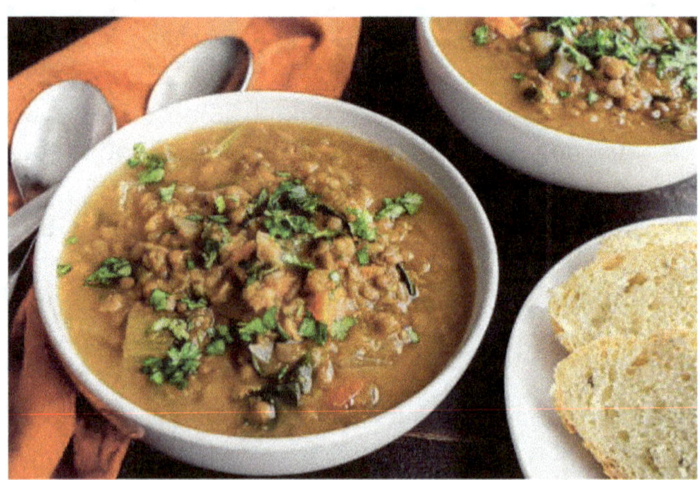

Ingredients:

For Lentil Soup:

- One tablespoon of olive oil.
- One medium onion, chopped.
- Two carrots, peeled and sliced
- Two celery stalks, chopped
- Two garlic cloves, minced
- 1 cup brown lentils, washed
- 4 cups veggie broth.
- 1 (14.5 oz) can of chopped tomatoes, undrained
- One teaspoon of dried thyme.
- ½ teaspoon ground cumin
- ¼ teaspoon red pepper flakes (optional)
- 4 cups of kale, coarsely chopped
- Add salt and freshly ground black pepper to taste.
- For Whole Wheat Bread (Makes One Loaf):
- 1 ½ cups heated water (105°F - 115°F)
- One tablespoon of active dry yeast.
- One tablespoon of honey or brown sugar.
- Three tablespoons olive oil.
- 3 ½ cups whole wheat flour, with extra for dusting.
- 1 ½ teaspoon salt.

Instructions:

1. Prepare the lentil soup:
- Bring the olive oil to medium heat in a big saucepan or Dutch oven. Add the chopped onions,

carrots, and celery. Sauté for 5-7 minutes or until tender and transparent.

- Stir in the minced garlic and simmer for another minute, allowing the garlic to unleash its aroma.
- Add the rinsed brown lentils, vegetable broth, chopped tomatoes (with juices), dried thyme, cumin, and red pepper flakes (optional). Season with a touch of salt and pepper.
- Bring to a boil, then decrease the heat to low, cover, and cook for 20-25 minutes until lentils are soft but still hold their form.

2. Prepare the whole wheat bread While the soup simmers (optional).

- Add warm water, yeast, and honey (or brown sugar) in a large mixing dish. Stir gently to dissolve the yeast and sugar. Allow the mixture to settle for 5–10 minutes or until bubbly and active.
- Mix in olive oil and 3 cups whole wheat flour. Mix until shaggy dough forms. Combine the remaining ½ cup flour and salt. Knead the dough on a lightly floured surface for 5-7 minutes or until it's smooth and elastic. If the dough seems too sticky, add a bit more flour.
- Area the dough in a greased basin and cover it with plastic wrap. Allow to rise in a warm area for 1-1 ½ hours or until doubled in size.

3. Back to Soup:

- Once the lentils are soft, add the chopped kale. Cook for 2-3 minutes or until the kale has wilted and softened.
- Taste the soup and season with salt and pepper as required.

4. Final touches:

- If you want to create whole wheat bread, preheat the oven to 375°F (190°C). Grease the loaf pan. After the dough has risen, punch it down and form it into a loaf. Place the bread in the prepared pan and bake for 30-35 minutes, until golden brown.
- Spoon the lentil soup into bowls while the bread is baking (or if you did not prepare bread).

5. Serve and Enjoy!

- Enjoy your hot lentil soup with a hefty piece of warm whole wheat bread to dip. Garnish your soup with a drizzle of olive oil, a freshly chopped parsley sprinkle, or a squeeze of lemon juice to add brightness.

Tips:

- Leftover lentil soup may be refrigerated in an airtight container for up to three days. Reheat gently on the burner before serving.

- Mix a portion of the cooked soup with an immersion blender before adding the kale to make a creamier soup.
- If you don't have brown lentils, you may use green lentils. Green lentils cook quicker, so adjust accordingly.
- Reduce the cooking time appropriately (approximately 5 minutes).
- This dish is readily tailored to your dietary requirements. Delete the honey and brown sugar from the bread recipe for a vegan variant and replace them with olive oil. You may also use veggie broth in the soup, and make sure your bread is vegan-certified.
- Add a spoonful of tomato paste to the soup mix and the chopped tomatoes for a fuller taste profile.

This lentil soup with kale is an excellent foundation for modification. Feel free to experiment with various veggies. Roasted red peppers, sliced mushrooms, or a handful of frozen peas may all provide variety and taste. Embrace Comfort and Goodness:

This lentil soup with kale and whole wheat bread is a hearty and fulfilling supper. It exemplifies how tasty cuisine can be healthy. This meal in your diet supplies your body with critical nutrients such as protein, iron, fibre, and fibreamins, all of which promote a healthy uterus and overall well-being. So, assemble your loved ones, prepare this soothing food, and enjoy the warmth and deliciousness in every mouthful!

4.3 Mediterranean Chickpea Salad With Sun-Dried Tomatoes

This colourful chickpea salad will transport you to the Mediterranean. This salad, packed with protein-rich chickpeas, savoury sun-dried tomatoes, and a symphony of fresh veggies, is a pleasant burst of taste and texture. It is not only delicious, but it also provides your body with critical nutrients that support a healthy uterus. Let's look at how to make this sunshine-filled meal ideal for a light lunch, refreshing side dish, or protein-packed vegetarian main course.

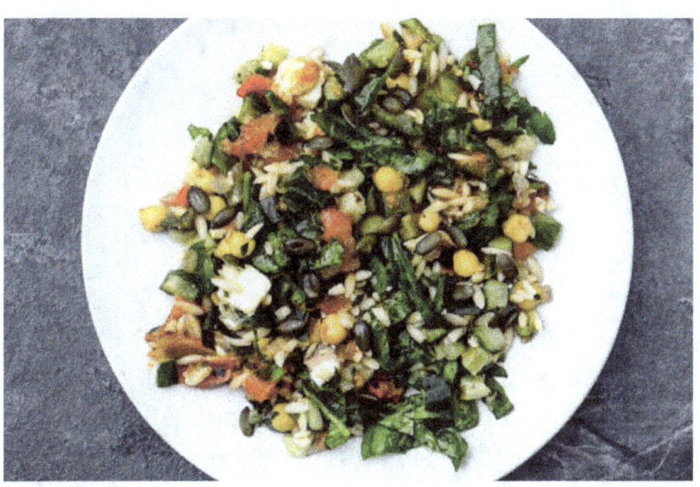

Ingredients:

For the salad:

- 1 (15-ounce) can of chickpeas, drained and rinsed
- One sliced cucumber (seeded, if preferred)
- One red bell pepper, chopped
- One red onion, finely chopped
- ½ cup crumbled feta cheese.
- ¼ cup chopped fresh parsley.
- ¼ cup chopped fresh mint.
- ¼ cup pitted and halved Kalamata olives (optional)

For the dressing:

- ¼ cup extra virgin olive oil.
- Two teaspoons of lemon juice.
- One tablespoon of red wine vinegar.
- One tablespoon chopped fresh oregano (or one teaspoon dried oregano)
- One garlic clove, minced
- ½ teaspoon dried thyme.
- A pinch of red pepper flakes (optional)
- Add salt and freshly ground black pepper to taste.

Instructions:

Prepare the salad ingredients.
1. In a large bowl, mix the drained and rinsed chickpeas, diced cucumber, diced red bell pepper, finely chopped red onion, crumbled feta cheese, chopped fresh parsley, chopped fresh mint, and halved kalamata olives (if using).

Prepare the dressing:

1. In a separate bowl, combine extra virgin olive oil, lemon juice, red wine vinegar, fresh oregano (or dried oregano), minced garlic clove, dried thyme, and a pinch of red pepper flakes (optional)—season with salt and freshly ground black pepper to taste.

Assemble, and enjoy!

1. In a large bowl, combine the chickpeas and vegetables. Pour the dressing over them. Gently toss all ingredients to ensure they are uniformly coated.
2. Taste and season with salt and pepper as required.
3. Serve the salad cold or at room temperature.

Tips:

- For a creamier salad, mash approximately ¼ cup of the chickpeas with a fork before adding them to the bowl. This will generate a thicker texture that can better retain the dressing.
- If you don't have fresh herbs, use one teaspoon of dried parsley and ½ teaspoon of dried mint for the chopped fresh herbs.
- Refrigerate leftovers in an airtight jar for up to three days. The flavours may develop even more overnight, making the salad even more delicious the following day!

A Symphony of Flavors and Nutrients:

This Mediterranean chickpea salad with sun-dried tomatoes is a beautiful and nutritious addition to your uterine-healthy diet. It's a gorgeous and savoury meal that will fuel your body while pleasing your taste senses! Packed with protein from chickpeas, healthy fats from olive oil and sun-dried tomatoes, and critical vitamins and minerals from veggies, this salad delivers a well-rounded variety of nutrients that may help a healthy reproductive system. So, grab your ingredients, release your inner chef, and prepare this sunshine-filled salad for a beautiful and healthful supper!

Chapter 5: Satisfying Main Courses

5.1 Salmon with Roasted Brussels Sprouts and Quinoa

This sheet-pan supper is a symphony of tastes and textures, overflowing with omega-3-rich salmon, crunchy roasted Brussels sprouts, and fluffy quinoa. It's a comprehensive and balanced meal that's very delectable and fills your body with critical nutrients for a healthy uterus. Let's go into producing this healthful cuisine, suitable for a weekday supper or a healthy lunch prep choice.

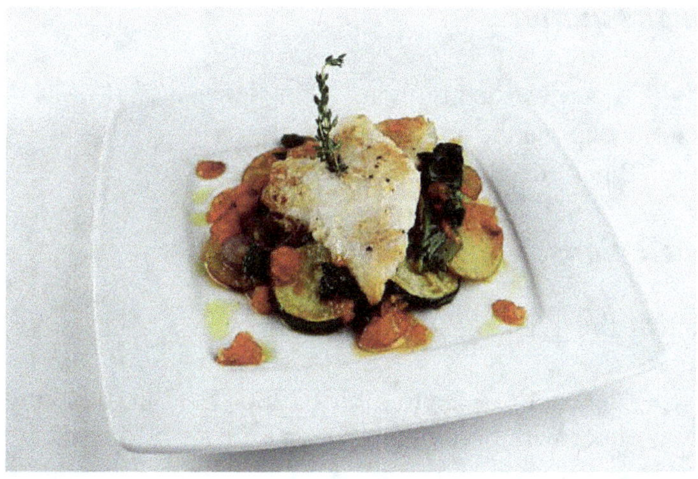

Ingredients:

For the Salmon:

- 2 (6 ounces) salmon fillets, skin-on
- One tablespoon of olive oil.
- One tablespoon of lemon juice.
- ½ teaspoon dried dill.
- Add salt and freshly ground black pepper to taste.

For the roasted Brussels sprouts:

- 1 pound of Brussels sprouts, cut and halved
- One tablespoon of olive oil.
- ½ teaspoon dried thyme.
- Add salt and freshly ground black pepper to taste.

For the quinoa:

- ½ cup washed quinoa.
- 1 cup water.
- Pinch of salt.

Instructions:

Preheat the oven.

1. Preheat the oven to 400 °F (200 °C). Line a baking sheet with parchment paper for easy cleaning.

Prepare the salmon:

1. Pat the salmon fillets dry with paper towels. Combine olive oil, lemon juice, and dried dill in a small bowl—season with salt and pepper. Brush the prepared marinade liberally onto the salmon fillets.

Prepare the Brussels sprouts:

1. Toss halved Brussels sprouts with olive oil, dried thyme, salt, and pepper. Spread them equally on one side of the prepared baking sheet.

Combine the quinoa:

1. Mix the rinsed quinoa, water, and a touch of salt in a small saucepan. Bring to a boil over medium heat. Reduce the heat 4 to low, cover the pan, and cook for 15-20 minutes or until the quinoa is fully cooked and fluffy. Set aside, lid on, to keep heated.

Assemble the baking sheet.

1. Place the marinated salmon fillets on the opposite half of the baking sheet, next to the Brussels sprouts. To ensure consistent cooking, arrange everything in a single layer.

Roast to perfection:

1. Bake for 15-20 minutes until the salmon is flaky and opaque in the middle and the Brussels sprouts are tender and slightly crunchy.

Plate and enjoy!

1. Divide the cooked quinoa into two dishes. Top each plate with a baked salmon fillet and plenty of crispy Brussels sprouts.

Tips:

- To test for doneness, lightly press the middle of the salmon fillet with a fork. If it flakes readily, it is fully cooked.
- You may cook quinoa using vegetable broth instead of water for a more tasty result. This will provide an additional layer of delicious delight.
- Feel free to modify the veggies! Chopped broccoli florets, asparagus spears, or sliced zucchini would make excellent additions to this sheet-pan supper.
- Refrigerate leftovers in an airtight jar for up to three days. Heat gently in the oven or microwave before serving.

A nutritional powerhouse.

This salmon with roasted Brussels sprouts and quinoa is a well-balanced meal that provides your body with essential nutrients. Salmon has a high concentration of omega-3 fatty acids necessary for hormonal balance and reproductive health. The Brussels sprouts provide vitamins and fibre, while the quinoa includes protein and complex carbs for sustained energy. Preheat your oven, assemble your ingredients, and prepare this delicious and nutritious recipe for a filling and healthy supper!

5.2 Curried Chickpea Stew with Sweet Potato.

This colourful stew combines toasty spices, creamy coconut milk, and soft veggies. This delectable recipe, packed with protein-rich chickpeas and fibre-filled sweet potato, will take your taste senses on a pleasurable trip while providing your body with essential nutrients for a healthy uterus. Let's look at how to make this fragrant curry, which is ideal for a relaxing night or a delicious midweek supper.

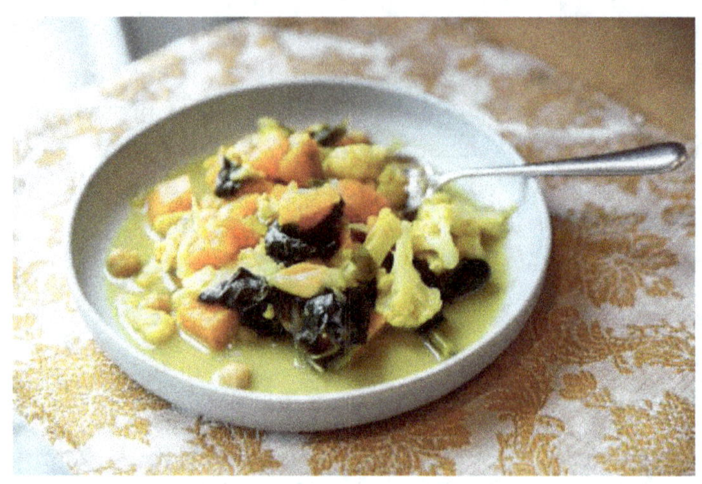

Ingredients:

For the stew:

- One tablespoon of olive oil.
- One medium onion, chopped.
- Two garlic cloves, minced
- One tablespoon of grated ginger.
- One teaspoon of curry powder.
- ½ teaspoon of turmeric powder.
- ½ teaspoon of ground cumin
- ¼ teaspoon of chilli powder (optional)
- 1 (15 oz) can of chopped tomatoes, undrained
- 1 (13.5 oz) can of coconut milk, full-fat or light.
- 1 cup veggie broth.
- 1 (15-ounce) can of chickpeas, drained and rinsed

- One big sweet potato, peeled and sliced into 1-inch chunks.
- One cup chopped spinach or kale.
- One tablespoon of chopped fresh cilantro (optional).
- Add salt and freshly ground black pepper to taste.
- For serving (optional)
- Cooked rice or quinoa
- Naan bread

Instructions:

Warm up the spices:
- Bring the olive oil to medium heat in a big saucepan or Dutch oven. Cook for 5-7 minutes until the onion is transparent.
- Introduce the aromatics.
- Stir in the minced garlic and grated ginger. Cook for another minute, allowing the pleasant scents to spread.

Unlock Curry Flavors:

- Combine the curry powder, turmeric powder, cumin, and chilli powder (if using). Sauté for 30 seconds, stirring regularly, to toast the spices and bring out their nuances.
- Bring it together:
- Pour in the chopped tomatoes (with liquids), coconut milk, and vegetable broth. Stir until combined and bring to a boil.

Welcome, Chickpeas and Sweet Potato:

- Combine the drained and rinsed chickpeas with the cubed sweet potato. Increase the heat slightly and return the mixture to a simmer.

Let the Flavors Mingle:

- Cover the saucepan, decrease the heat to low, and cook for 15-20 minutes or until the sweet potatoes are cooked.

Embrace the Green:

- Add the chopped spinach or kale and simmer for 2-3 minutes or until wilted.

Season and garnish (optional):

- Season the stew with salt and freshly ground black pepper to taste. Garnish with chopped fresh cilantro (optional) to add brightness.

Serve and Enjoy!

- Spoon the curried chickpea stew into dishes. Serve with cooked rice or quinoa and heated naan bread (optional) to dip.

Tips:

- For a thicker stew, use a fork to mash some of the chickpeas against the edge of the pot before adding the spinach or kale. This produces a thicker consistency.
- If you like a hotter stew, include a sprinkle of red pepper flakes with the other spices in step 3.
- Feel free to modify the veggies! Chopped carrots, bell peppers, or a handful of green beans would make excellent additions to this savoury curry.
- Refrigerate leftovers in an airtight jar for up to three days. Reheat gently on the burner before serving.

A Symphony of Flavor and Well-Being:

This curried chickpea and sweet potato stew is a tasty and nutritious addition to your uterine-healthy diet. It's a harmonious blend of spicy spices, creamy coconut milk, and soft veggies. Chickpeas are high in protein and fibre, while sweet potatoes include vitamin A and antioxidants. The curry powder, turmeric, and cumin all have anti-inflammatory effects, making this meal tasty and good for general health. So, go on an aromatic trip, make this delicious stew, and fill your body with a taste of comfort and goodness!

5.3 Stir-fried Chicken with Broccoli and Brown Rice

This colourful stir-fry is a symphony of textures and tastes, packed with lean protein from chicken, crisp-tender broccoli florets, and nutty whole-grain brown rice. It's a fast and straightforward supper that tastes great and improves uterine health because of its well-rounded nutritional profile. Let's look at how to make this delicious stir-fry, ideal for a hectic evening or a nutritious lunch.

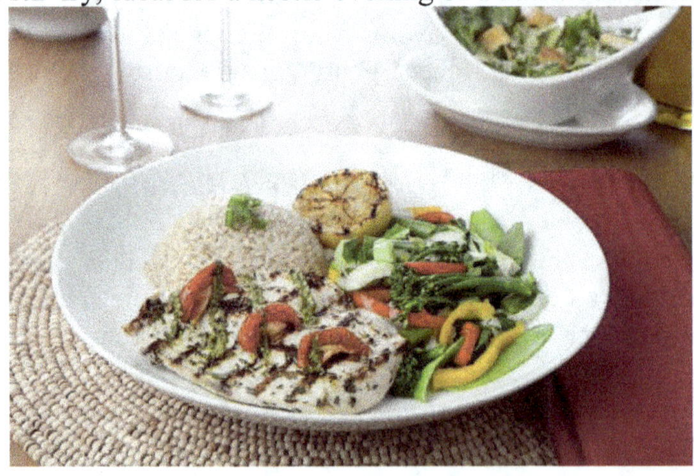

Ingredients:

For the stir-fry:

- One tablespoon of cornstarch.
- Two tablespoons soy sauce (or tamari for the gluten-free version)
- One tablespoon of honey.
- One tablespoon of rice vinegar.
- One teaspoon of sesame oil.
- ½ teaspoon grated ginger.
- A pinch of garlic powder.
- A pinch of red pepper flakes (optional)
- 1 pound of boneless, skinless chicken breasts or thighs, thinly sliced
- One tablespoon of vegetable oil.
- One cup of broccoli florets.
- ½ cup chopped red bell pepper (optional)
- ¼ cup chopped onion (optional)
- ¼ cup sliced carrots (optional)
- Two cups of cooked brown rice.
- For serving (optional)
- I toasted sesame seeds.
- Chopped green onion

Instructions:

Prepare the sauce.

- In a small mixing bowl, combine cornstarch, soy sauce (or tamari), honey, rice vinegar, sesame oil, grated ginger, garlic powder, and red pepper flakes (if used). Set aside.
- Marinate the chicken.
- Put the thinly sliced chicken in a medium bowl. Pour half of the prepared sauce over the chicken and toss to coat evenly. Marinate for at least 15 or 30 minutes for a richer taste.
- Cook the brown rice (optional)
- If you haven't previously cooked brown rice, follow the package directions. While the chicken marinates, make your rice.

Heat the wok:

- Heat the vegetable oil in a big wok or pan over high heat. (If you don't have a wok, a big frying pan works well.)
- Sear the chicken.
- Add the marinated chicken when the oil is heated and shimmering (discard any remaining marinade). Stir fry for 3-4 minutes or until the chicken is fully cooked and golden brown. Remove the cooked chicken from the pan and place it on a platter.

Welcome, Vegetables:

- Add the broccoli florets, red bell pepper (if using), onion, and carrots to the wok. Stir-fry the veggies for 2-3 minutes or until crisp-tender.
- Bring back the chicken and sauce.
- Pour the leftover sauce into the pan with the veggies. Bring to a boil, then cook for another minute or until the sauce thickens slightly.

Reunite the Chicken and Stir-Fry:

- Return the chicken to the skillet and stir with the veggies and sauce.

Assemble, and enjoy!

- Divide the cooked brown rice onto two plates. Top each plate with the stir-fry mixture. Garnish with toasted sesame seeds and chopped green onions (optional) to add flavour and colour.

Tips:

- Cut the chicken into thin strips against the grain to ensure it cooks evenly.
- If your stir-fry seems too dry, add a dash of water or chicken stock while cooking the veggies.
- Feel free to modify the veggies! Chopped snow peas, zucchini slices, or baby corn would make excellent additions to this stir-fry.

- Refrigerate leftovers in an airtight jar for up to three days. Reheat gently in a pan or microwave before serving.

A nutritious weeknight delight:

This chicken stir-fry with broccoli and brown rice is a tasty and healthy dish for hectic weeknights. The chicken is a fantastic source of lean protein, while the broccoli contains vitamins and fibre. Whole-grain brown rice provides complex carbs for lasting energy. This meal is a well-rounded and pleasant choice that may help maintain a healthy uterus by encouraging hormonal balance and general well-being. So take your work, collect your ingredients, and stir-fry your way to a delicious and nutritious lunch!

Chapter 6: Comforting Soups & Stews.

6.1 Creamy Butternut Squash Soup With Ginger

This colourful soup is a harmonious blend of creamy texture and seasonal tastes. This soothing recipe, packed with roasted butternut squash, ginger for warmth, and a dash of sweetness, feeds your body while delighting your taste senses. It's an excellent accompaniment to a cold day or a delicious appetizer for a lovely evening.

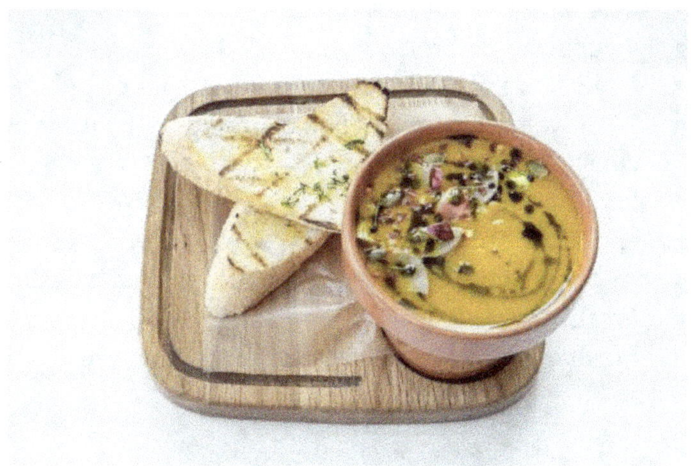

Ingredients:

For the roast squash:

- One medium butternut squash (about. 3 pounds), peeled, seeded, and diced.
- One tablespoon of olive oil.
- ½ teaspoon dried thyme.
- Add salt and freshly ground black pepper to taste.

For the soup:

- One tablespoon of olive oil.
- One medium onion, chopped.
- Two garlic cloves, minced
- One tablespoon of grated ginger.
- 4 cups veggie broth.
- 1 (13.5 oz) can of coconut milk, full-fat or light.
- 1 cup water (more or less according to the desired consistency)
- ½ teaspoon ground cumin
- A pinch of red pepper flakes (optional)
- Add salt and freshly ground black pepper to taste.
- Freshly grated nutmeg (optional).
- Fresh cilantro or parsley, chopped (for garnish)

Instructions:

Roast the butternut squash.

- Preheat the oven to 400 °F (200 °C). Line a baking sheet with parchment paper for easy cleaning.
- Combine the cubed butternut squash, olive oil, dried thyme, salt, and pepper in a large mixing bowl. Spread the squash equally on the prepared baking sheet.
- Roast for 25-30 minutes, or until the squash is soft and lightly browned, rotating the cubes halfway through.
- Sauté the aromatics.
- While the squash roasts, warm the olive oil in a large saucepan or Dutch oven over medium heat. Cook for 5-7 minutes until the onion is transparent.

Introduce ginger and garlic:

- Stir in the minced garlic and grated ginger. Cook for another minute, allowing the pleasant scents to spread.
- Bring on the broth and coconut milk!
- Pour in the veggie broth and coconut milk. Bring to a simmer.

Welcome, Roasted Squash:

- Add the roasted butternut squash to the saucepan and any juices from the baking sheet.

Blend till creamy perfection:

- Puree the soup with an immersion blender or in batches until smooth and creamy. You may also use a potato masher to get a more rustic texture.
- Season and simmer.
- Stir in the ground cumin, red pepper flakes (if using), salt, and pepper. Taste and adjust spices as needed. Simmer for another 5 minutes to let the flavours mingle.

Garnish and enjoy!

- Ladle the velvety butternut squash soup into individual bowls. Garnish with freshly grated nutmeg (optional) and chopped fresh parsley or cilantro for a vibrant touch. Serve with warm, crusty bread for dipping.

Tips:

- To save time, instead of roasting the butternut squash, sauté it with the onions until tender before adding the stock. However, roasting imparts a more profound and richer taste to the soup.

- Add more water or stock for consistency if your soup seems too thick.
- Feel free to change the spices! A pinch of ground coriander or a dash of turmeric would welcome diversity to the taste profile.
- Refrigerate leftovers in an airtight jar for up to three days. Reheat gently on the burner before serving.

Comforting Embrace in a Bowl

This creamy butternut squash soup with ginger is a tasty and nutritious addition to your diet. It's a lovely orange symphony of tastes that soothes your body and spirit. Butternut squash is high in vitamin A and antioxidants, while ginger has anti-inflammatory properties. This cosy soup is an excellent method to fuel your body and boost overall health. Preheat your oven, assemble your ingredients, and prepare this tasty creamy dish for a delicious and filling lunch!

6.2 Lentil And Vegetable Soup with Whole Wheat Noodles

This rustic lentil and vegetable soup will wrap you in a warm hug. This symphony of textures and tastes is not only delightful, but it also provides your body with critical nutrients. Let's create a culinary tapestry using protein-rich lentils, a colourful array of veggies, and hearty whole-wheat noodles. This dish is ideal for a relaxing night in, a delicious lunch, or a nutritious meal prep for busy weekdays.

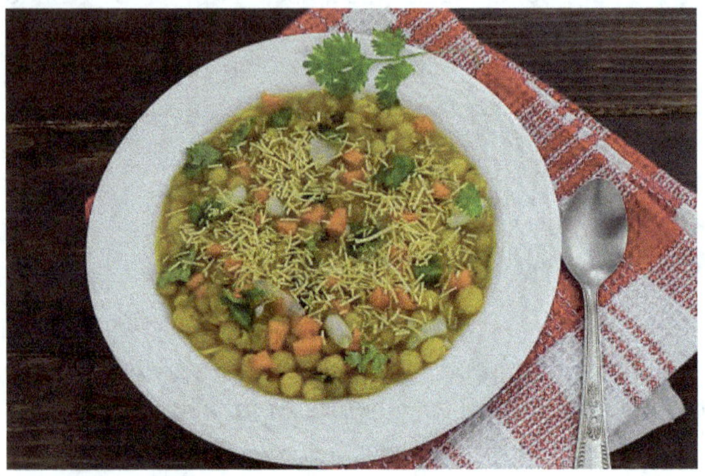

Ingredients:

For the broth:

- One tablespoon of olive oil.
- One medium onion, chopped.
- Two carrots, peeled and sliced
- Two celery stalks, chopped
- One clove of garlic, minced
- 8 cups veggie broth.
- One bay leaf.
- Add salt and freshly ground black pepper to taste.

For the soup:

- 1 cup brown lentils, washed
- 1 (14.5 oz) can of chopped tomatoes, undrained
- One cup of chopped broccoli florets.
- 1/2 cup chopped green beans.
- ½ cup frozen peas.
- Four cups of cooked whole wheat noodles.

Optional additions:

- Chopped kale or spinach (for more greens)
- Diced zucchini or yellow squash (for extra summer tastes)
- Dried herbs such as thyme, oregano, or rosemary (for an earthy flavour)

Instructions:

Create the Base:

- Bring the olive oil to medium heat in a big saucepan or Dutch oven. Add the chopped onions, carrots, and celery. Sauté for 5-7 minutes or until tender and transparent. Add the minced garlic and heat for another minute, allowing the delicious smells to develop.

Build the broth:

- Pour in the veggie broth, then add the bay leaf—season with salt and pepper to taste. Bring the mixture to a boil, decrease the heat to low, cover, and cook for 15 minutes.

Welcome, Lentils:

- Add the washed brown lentils to the boiling stock. Cook for 20-25 minutes until the lentils are cooked but hold their form.

Introduce the vegetables:

- Add the diced tomatoes (with liquids), chopped broccoli florets, green beans, and frozen peas. Increase the heat slightly and return the soup to a simmer. Cook for another 5-7 minutes until the veggies are soft and crisp.

Unite the Noodles:

- Gently fold the cooked whole wheat noodles, ensuring they are uniformly distributed throughout the soup.
- A touch of green (optional)
- Add chopped kale or spinach and simmer for another minute or until wilted.

Season and Savour:

- Taste the soup and season with salt and pepper as required. Remove the bay leaf before serving.
- Celebrate the Rustic Delight!
- Spoon the steamed lentils and vegetable soup into dishes. This hearty recipe is delicious but may also be served with crusty whole-wheat bread for dipping.

Tips:

- Refrigerate leftovers in an airtight jar for up to three days. Reheat gently on the burner before serving.
- To make a creamier soup, use an immersion blender to partly purée some of the cooked lentils and veggies before adding the noodles.
- Feel free to experiment with various veggies! Chopped mushrooms, bell peppers, or even a handful of corn kernels would make excellent additions to this rustic soup.
- This dish is readily tailored to your dietary requirements. For a vegan version, avoid using vegetable broth containing animal ingredients and ensure your whole wheat noodles are vegan-certified.

A Nourishing tapestry for your well-being:

This lentil and vegetable soup with whole wheat noodles is more than a tasty dinner; it's a tapestry of vital nutrients for your health. Lentils are high in protein and fibre, while veggies include a variety of vitamins and minerals. Whole wheat noodles provide complex carbs for prolonged energy. So grab your ingredients, turn on the stove, and prepare this cosy and nourishing dish to enjoy the simple joys of a nutritious and delectable supper.

6.3 Hearty Chicken Noodle Soup.

There's a reason chicken noodle soup is a favourite comfort food: it's warm, filling, and flavorful. This hearty variation enhances the original dish with a thick homemade broth and various healthy veggies. It's the ideal dinner for soothing a sore throat, warming up on a cold day, or enjoying a filling and nutritious dish.

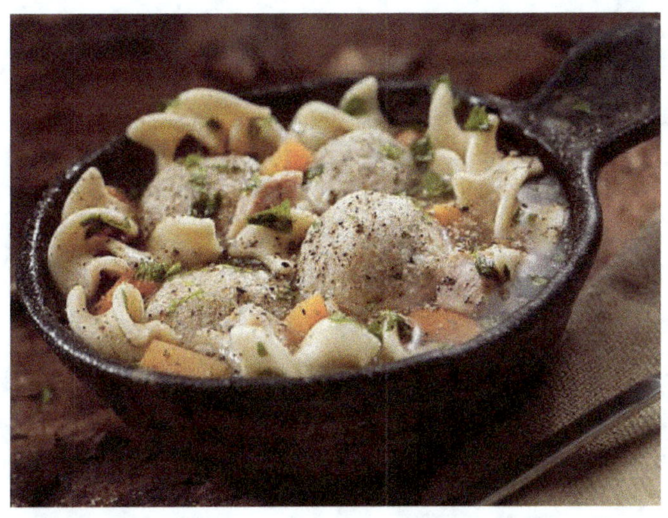

Ingredients:

For the broth:

- One chicken (about 3-4 lbs) is chopped into pieces (breast, thighs, wings, and drumsticks).
- One onion, peeled and quartered
- Two carrots peeled and coarsely sliced.
- Two celery stalks, coarsely diced.
- Three garlic cloves, crushed
- One teaspoon of dried thyme.
- One bay leaf.
- Eight glasses of water.
- Add salt and freshly ground black pepper to taste.
- For the soup:
- Two tablespoons olive oil.

- One medium onion, chopped.
- Two carrots, peeled and sliced
- Two celery stalks, chopped
- 4 cups chopped mixed veggies (such as peas, corn, and green beans)
- 8 cups chicken broth (from step one or store-bought low-sodium broth)
- 4 cups cooked egg noodles (or your chosen noodle kind)
- Chopped fresh parsley (optional for garnish).

Instructions:

Make a flavorful broth:

1. Add the chicken, quartered onion, carrots, celery, crushed garlic cloves, dried thyme, bay leaf, and water in a large saucepan—Season well with salt and pepper. Bring to a boil, then decrease heat and simmer for 1-1/2 to 2 hours, or until the chicken is fully cooked and the veggies are soft.
2. Strain and shred the chicken.
3. Remove the saucepan from the heat and gently remove the chicken pieces. Set aside to cool somewhat. Strain the broth into a clean saucepan and discard the sediments.
4. When the chicken is cold enough to handle, shred the flesh from the bones and discard the skin and bones.
5. Sauté the vegetables.

6. Bring the olive oil to medium heat in a big saucepan or Dutch oven. Add the chopped onion, carrots, and celery. Sauté for 5-7 minutes or until tender and transparent.

Welcome, Broth and Chicken:

1. Pour the strained chicken broth into the saucepan containing the sautéed veggies. Bring to a simmer. Mix in the shredded chicken and mixed veggies.

Noodle time!

2. Stir in the cooked egg noodles (or your choice of noodle) to the boiling soup. Cook for another 3-5 minutes until the noodles are cooked through.
3. A touch of freshness (optional)
4. Sprinkle chopped fresh parsley over each portion before serving to add a bit of brightness.

Serve and Enjoy!

- Ladle the boiling chicken noodle soup into bowls. This warm recipe is delicious but may also be served with crusty bread for dipping or a side salad to make a complete meal.

Tips:

- Refrigerate leftovers in an airtight jar for up to three days. Reheat gently on the burner before serving.
- For added flavour, roast the broth vegetables (carrots, celery, and onion) in a preheated oven at 400°F (200°C) for 20-25 minutes before adding them to the pot.
- This recipe may be readily customized! Feel free to include your favourite veggies, such as mushrooms, zucchini, or spinach.
- You may use leftover rotisserie chicken to reduce cooking time. Shred the cooked chicken and mix it into the soup in step 4.

A Nourishing embrace in a bowl:

This hearty chicken noodle soup is more than a great comfort dish; it's a cosy hug in a bowl. The homemade chicken broth is flavorful and nutritious, and the veggies and noodles include necessary vitamins, minerals, and complex carbs. So collect your ingredients, boil the broth compassionately, and prepare this traditional recipe to feed your body and spirit.

Part 3: Sweet Treats to Enjoy

Chapter 7: Guiltless Desserts and Snacks (6 Recipes)

7.1 Baked apples with cinnamon and walnuts.

Enjoy the flavour of autumn with this delectable dish of baked apples. Bursting with fragrant spices, the apples' sweetness blends with the delightful crunch of walnuts to create a symphony of textures and aromas. This simple but gorgeous dessert is ideal for a relaxing night, a delectable after-dinner treat, or a nutritious and filling snack.

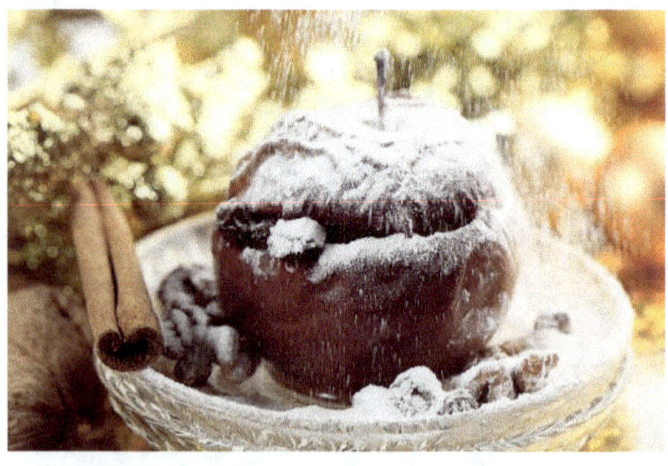

Ingredients:

- Four medium apples (Gala, Honeycrisp, or Braeburn)
- ¼.cup chopped walnuts.
- ¼ cup brown sugar (packaged)
- Two tablespoons melted butter
- One teaspoon of ground cinnamon.
- ¼ teaspoon of ground nutmeg (optional)
- 1/8 teaspoon of ground ginger (optional)
- Pinch of salt.
- ¼ cup of chopped raisins (optional).
- Vanilla ice cream or whipped cream for serving (optional).

Instructions:

Preheat the oven.

- Preheat the oven to 375°F (190° C). Lightly grease or line a baking dish with parchment paper to make cleaning easier.

Prepare the apples:

- Wash and dry the apples. A melon baller or a tiny spoon is used to core the apples from the top, leaving the bottoms intact. This will keep the filling from leaking out while baking.

Craft the Filling:

- Mix the chopped walnuts, brown sugar, melted butter, cinnamon, nutmeg (if used), ginger (if used), and a touch of salt in a small bowl. Mix well to form a fragrant crumble.
- Stuff and bake.
- Distribute the crumble filling equally among the cored apples. If using raisins, carefully push them into the filling. Place the packed apples in the prepared baking dish.

Baking to perfection:

- Bake the apples for 30-40 minutes or until fork-tender and the filling bubbling.

A touch of indulgence (optional):

- During the final 5 minutes of baking, sprinkle a spoonful of maple syrup or honey over the tops of the cooked apples for an extra luscious finish.

Serve and Enjoy!

- Let the cooked apples cool slightly before serving. Transfer to plates or bowls. Serve warm with a dollop of vanilla ice cream or whipped cream (optional) for a delicious and filling dessert.

Tips:

- To achieve consistent baking, use apples of comparable sizes.
- If the apples seem dry during baking, add a tablespoon or two of water or apple juice to the bottom of the baking dish.
- Feel free to experiment with various fillings! Chopped dried cranberries, pecans, or chopped dates would all make great additions to this recipe.
- Refrigerate leftovers in an airtight jar for up to three days. Reheat gently in the microwave or oven before serving.

Celebration of Autumn Flavors:

Baked apples with cinnamon and walnuts celebrate the scents of autumn. They are not only tasty but also nutritious and fulfilling dessert options. Apples are high in fibre and vitamin C, while walnuts include healthy fats and protein. So, preheat your oven, grab your ingredients, and make this delicious dessert to celebrate the spirit of autumn while nourishing your body with seasonal deliciousness!

7.2 Dark Chocolate Avocado Mousse.

This dish is a delicious take on the traditional chocolate mousse, with a rich and creamy texture and an unexpected healthful twist! Made with ripe avocados and luscious dark chocolate, this mousse is delicious and high in healthy fats and antioxidants. This dark chocolate avocado mousse is ideal for a guilt-free pleasure or as a show-stopping dessert.

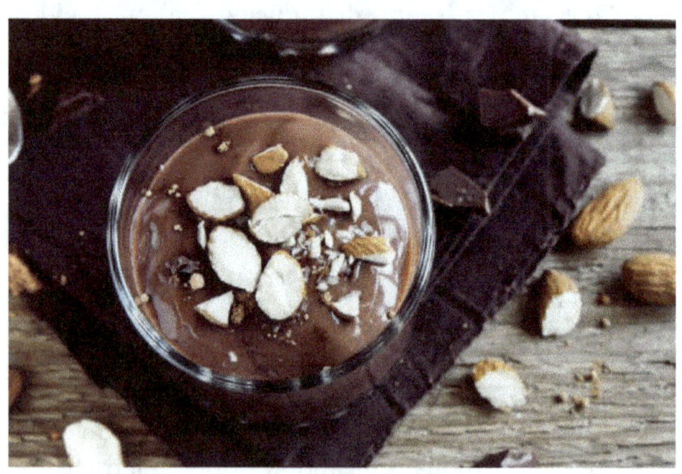

Ingredients:

- Two ripe avocados, halved, pitted and scooped.
- 4 ounces of dark chocolate (at least 60% cacao), melted (see choices below)
- ¼ cup unsweetened cocoa powder.
- 1/3 cup of maple syrup (or honey for a slightly different taste profile)
- 1/3 cup unsweetened almond milk (or your favourite plant-based milk).
- ½ teaspoon of vanilla essence.
- Pinch of salt.

Optional toppings:

- Whipped cream (dairy, coconut)
- Chocolate shavings
- Fresh berries
- Chopped nuts
- Melting methods for dark chocolate:

Double Boiler Method:
1. Fill a saucepan with a few inches of water.
2. Heat the water to a simmer.
3. Melt the chocolate in a separate heat-resistant bowl on top of the saucepan (but not in contact with the water), stirring occasionally until smooth.

Microwave Method: Put the chocolate in a microwave-safe bowl. Microwave at high power for 30-second intervals, stirring in between, until melted and smooth. Be careful not to overheat the chocolate, as it may burn.

Instructions:

Prepare the avocado:

- To achieve the creamiest texture, ensure that your avocados are perfectly ripe. Scoop the avocado flesh into a blender or food processor.
- Combine the creamy base:
- Pour the melted dark chocolate, cocoa powder, maple syrup (or honey), almond milk, vanilla

extract, and a pinch of salt into the blender or food processor with the avocado flesh.

Blend for Smooth Perfection:

- Blend until the mixture is smooth and creamy, scraping down the sides if necessary. Depending on your blender's power, this could take 30-60 seconds.

Taste and adjust (optional):

- Give the mousse a taste and adjust the sweetness and cocoa powder content as needed.

Divide and Chill:

- Divide the mousse evenly between two or three serving dishes. Cover and refrigerate for at least 2 hours or until chilled and set.

Time to Indulge!

- Remove the mousse from the refrigerator and garnish with your desired toppings (whipped cream, chocolate shavings, fresh berries, chopped nuts, or a combination).

Savour the Healthy Decadence!

- Dive into your creation and savour the rich and creamy texture of this delightful dark chocolate avocado mousse. Enjoy the guilt-free indulgence, knowing you're nourishing your body with healthy fats and antioxidants.

Tips:

- For a more decadent mousse, use dark chocolate with a higher cacao percentage (70% or higher).
- Add a tablespoon or two of additional almond milk to achieve your desired consistency if your mixture seems too thick.
- This mousse is best enjoyed chilled, but it can be stored in an airtight container in the refrigerator for up to 2 days. The flavour and texture may change slightly over time.

A Guilt-Free Celebration:

Dark chocolate avocado mousse is a celebration of healthy indulgence. It provides a rich and creamy dessert option that is satisfying and good for you. The avocados offer healthy fats and fibre, while the dark chocolate boasts antioxidants. So, gather your ingredients, embrace your inner chef, and create this delightful and decadent mousse to celebrate the goodness of healthy and flavorful treats!

7.3 Energy Balls with Dates, Nuts, and Seeds

These delightful energy balls are nature's answer to a convenient and healthy pick-me-up. Bursting with the sweetness of dates, the satisfying crunch of nuts and seeds, and packed with protein and fibre, these bite-sized treats are perfect for a pre-workout snack, an afternoon energy boost, or a healthy and satisfying sweet treat. This recipe is easily customizable to suit your taste preferences and dietary needs, making it a versatile and fun way to incorporate wholesome ingredients into your diet.

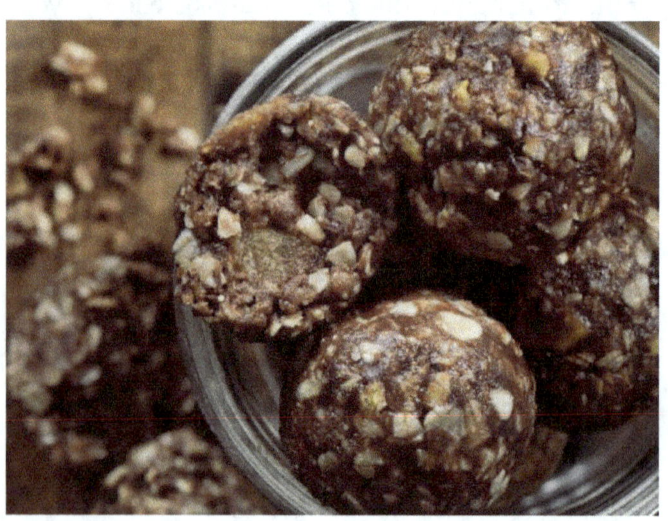

Ingredients:

Base:

- 1 cup pitted Medjool dates (about 15-20 dates)
- ½ cup rolled oats (or quick oats)
- ½ cup chopped nuts (such as almonds, cashews, peanuts, or a mixture)
- ¼ cup chopped seeds (such as chia seeds, flaxseeds, sunflower seeds, pumpkin seeds, or a mixture)
- Sweeteners and Flavorings (Optional):
- ¼ cup chopped dried fruit (such as raisins, cranberries, or chopped apricots)
- ¼ cup nut butter (such as almond butter, peanut butter, or cashew butter)
- One tablespoon of honey or maple syrup
- Half a teaspoon of crushed cinnamon
- ¼ teaspoon ground ginger
- Pinch of sea salt

Instructions:

Prepare the Dates:

- Ensure your dates are soft and pliable. Soak them in warm water for 10-15 minutes to soften if they are dry. Drain thoroughly before using.

Blend the Base:

- Combine the pitted dates, rolled oats, chopped nuts, and chopped seeds in a food processor. Pulse the mixture until it comes together, scraping down the sides as needed.

Incorporate Sweeteners and Flavorings (Optional):

- If using any optional ingredients like chopped dried fruit, nut butter, honey or maple syrup, spices, or salt, add them to the food processor at this point.

Achieve the Perfect Consistency:

- Continue to pulse and process the mixture until it reaches a sticky and cohesive consistency that can easily be pressed into balls. You may need to scrape down the sides a few times and pulse again to ensure everything is evenly incorporated.

From the Energy Balls:

- Wet your hands slightly to prevent sticking. Scoop about 1-2 tablespoons of the mixture and roll it into a ball between your palms. Gently press down to compact the ball. Repeat with the remaining mixture.

Optional Coating (Optional):

- For extra flavour and texture, you can roll the finished energy balls in additional toppings like shredded coconut, chopped nuts, cocoa powder, or hemp seeds.

Chill and Enjoy!

- Place the energy balls in a container with a lid and refrigerate for at least 30 minutes or until firm. This allows the flavours to meld and the dates to set.

Store and Savor:

- Store leftover energy balls in an airtight container in the refrigerator for up to 2 weeks.

Tips:

- If your mixture seems too dry after pulsing, add a tablespoon or two of water or additional softened dates to achieve the desired consistency.
- For a more intense nut or seed flavour, toast them lightly in a dry pan before adding them to the food processor.
- This recipe is easily adaptable to dietary needs. Use nut butter alternatives like sunflower seed butter or tahini for nut allergies. For a vegan

option, omit honey and ensure your chosen nut butter and other ingredients are vegan-certified.
- Feel free to experiment with different flavour combinations! Dried fruits like chopped mango or figs would add a delightful twist, while spices like cardamom or nutmeg can offer a warm and exotic touch.

Nature's Energy on the Go:

These date, nut, and seed energy balls are a delicious and convenient way to fuel your body with natural goodness. They are packed with essential nutrients, fibre, and healthy fats to energize you throughout the day. So, gather your ingredients, unleash your creativity, and create a batch of these delightful energy balls to enjoy whenever you need a natural pick-me-up!

Part 4: The Bigger Picture

Chapter 8: Lifestyle Habits for Optimal Uterine Health

8.1 Exercise and Movement

Exercise and movement are not just about burning calories or sculpting a physique; they are a vibrant symphony for your body and soul. It's a chance to celebrate the incredible machine that carries you through life, a way to express yourself freely, and a journey to discover a deeper connection with your inner strength and resilience.

Imagine your body as a magnificent orchestra—each muscle is a string, each bone is a percussion instrument, and your breath is the conductor. As you move, you create a symphony of motion. A brisk walk becomes a lively allegro, a yoga flow a graceful adagio, and a dance session a pulsating, rhythmic crescendo.

The Overture: Finding Your Movement Muse

The first step in this symphony is finding your movement muse. What ignites a spark of joy within you? Is it the exhilaration of a run in the crisp morning air, the meditative flow of tai chi, or the playful energy of a Zumba class? There's no right or wrong answer – the key is to discover activities that make you want to move and truly feel the music within your body.

The Crescendo: Embracing the Benefits

As you move, the benefits begin to unfold like a beautiful melody. Exercise strengthens your muscles, improves cardiovascular health, and boosts energy levels. It also acts as a powerful stress reliever, washing away tension and anxiety with each step, bend, or stretch. It can even enhance cognitive function and improve sleep quality, leaving you feeling sharper and more rested.

The Harmony: Celebrating Every Body

The beauty of movement lies in its inclusivity. There's no need to strive for a specific physique; the joy lies in celebrating the unique instrument that is your body. Whether you're tall or short, slender or firm, there's a movement symphony waiting to be composed.

The Intermission: Rest and Recovery

Just like a musical performance requires moments of silence for the music to resonate, your body needs time to rest and recover. Listen to your body's cues. Take rest days, stretch regularly, and prioritize Sleep. This allows your muscles to rebuild and your energy to replenish, ensuring you can return to your movement symphony feeling refreshed and ready to create new melodies.

The Grand Finale: A Lifelong Journey

Exercise and movement aren't a sprint; they're a lifelong journey of discovery. There will be days when motivation wanes, but remember the joy of movement, the connection with your body, and the symphony of benefits it brings. Let your inner conductor guide you, explore new genres of movement, and celebrate the incredible gift of being able to move, express yourself, and feel the vibrant rhythm of life coursing through you.

So, step onto the stage of your body, pick up your chosen instrument, and compose your movement symphony. Let your body sing, your muscles play, and your spirit soar as you celebrate the joy of movement and the magnificent power within you.

8.2 Stress Management Techniques

Conquering Chaos: Effective Techniques for Stress Management

Stress. It's a four-letter word that can wreak havoc on our minds, bodies, and overall well-being. But fear not, for within us lies the power to manage stress and cultivate inner peace. Here's a symphony of techniques to help you become a maestro of your emotional well-being:

The Calming Chorus: Mindfulness and Meditation

Mindfulness and meditation are powerful tools for quieting the storm of swirling thoughts and anxieties. By focusing on the present moment, your breath, and bodily sensations, you can detach from stressful situations and cultivate inner calm. Techniques like mindfulness meditation and deep breathing exercises can be practised anywhere, anytime, offering a quick and effective stress-relieving pause.

The Rhythmic Release: Exercise and Movement

Exercise isn't just about physical fitness; it's a potent stress reliever. Physical activity releases endorphins, the body's natural feel-good chemicals, which combat stress hormones and elevate mood. From a brisk walk or a natural jog to a dance session in your living room, find an activity that gets your heart rate up and your body moving. As you move, stress melts away, replaced by a sense of accomplishment and renewed energy.

The Restorative Melody: Sleep and Relaxation

When stress lingers, our bodies and minds struggle to cope. Prioritizing quality sleep becomes essential. Aim for 7-8 hours of restful Sleep each night. Establish a relaxing bedtime routine, create a sleep-conducive environment, and power down electronic devices before bed. Additionally, relaxation techniques like progressive muscle relaxation or guided imagery can help ease tension and prepare you for a deep and restorative sleep.

The Supportive Harmony: Social Connection and Support

We are social creatures, and strong social connections are a powerful buffer against stress. Talking to a trusted friend, family member, or therapist can provide emotional support and a safe space to vent your frustrations. Laughter is also a powerful stress reliever, so don't underestimate the power of spending time with loved ones who make you smile.

The Calibrating Notes: Time Management and Boundaries

Do you need help with a never-ending to-do list? Effective time management is crucial for reducing stress. Prioritize tasks, create realistic schedules, and delegate when possible. Setting boundaries is equally important. Learn to say "no" to requests that drain your energy and establish clear boundaries between work and personal life.

The Uplifting Tempo: Healthy Habits and Self-Care

Taking care of oneself is not a luxury; it's a need in the battle against stress. Nourish your body with a balanced diet of fruits, vegetables, and whole grains. Avoid excessive coffee and alcohol since they might worsen anxiety. Engage in things you like, whether reading, spending time in nature, listening to music, or following a hobby. Prioritize self-care routines that offer you delight and encourage relaxation.

Remember: Stress management is a process, not a destination. Experiment with various ways, discover what works best for you, and be gentle to yourself along the journey. By implementing these stress-busting tactics into your life, you can become a maestro of your well-being, creating a symphony of serenity and resilience in the face of life's obstacles.

Calming the Inner Storm: Effective Techniques for Stress Management

Stress. It's a constant companion in our fast-paced world, a persistent undercurrent that might threaten to take us under. But worry not because there are practical strategies to reduce stress and nurture inner calm.
Here's a toolkit loaded with methods to help you manage the storms of stress and discover moments of calm:

Mindfulness & Meditation:

- **Center Yourself:** Mindfulness activities like meditation help you become aware of the present moment without judgment. Take a few deep breaths, concentrate on your surroundings, and watch your thoughts and sensations without getting caught up in them.

- **Meditation Apps:** Numerous meditation apps provide guided meditation for stress relief. These guided trips help you concentrate your attention, quiet your mind, and encourage relaxation.

Body-Based Techniques:

- **Deep Breathing:** Deep, calm breaths induce the relaxation response in your body, counteracting the fight-or-flight reaction caused by stress.

- **Progressive Muscle Relaxation:** Tense and relax various muscle groups gradually, beginning with your toes and working your way up your body. This may reduce physical stress and create emotions of relaxation.

- **Yoga and Tai Chi** are mind-body disciplines that include gentle movements, deep breathing, and meditation. They may increase flexibility, lower stress hormones, and boost emotions of well-being.

Physical Activity:

- **Move Your Body:** Exercise is an effective stress reducer. Take a quick walk, go to the gym, or dance in your living room. Physical exercise causes the body to produce endorphins, natural feel-good chemicals that may significantly boost mood and decrease stress.

- **Connect with Nature:** Spending time in nature may relieve stress. Stroll in the park, go in the woods, or sit outdoors and listen to nature's noises.

Healthy Habits for Long-term Stress Management

- **Prioritize Sleep:** When well-rested, you're more prepared to deal with stress. Aim for 7-8 hours of good Sleep each night.

- **Healthy Diet:** Feed your body nourishing meals. Avoid processed meals, sweets, and caffeine since these might exacerbate stress symptoms.

- **Limit Screen Time:** Constant stimulation from electronic gadgets may lead to stress. Set aside some screen-free time each day to disengage and relax.

- **Positive Connections:** Having social support is essential for managing stress. Spend time with your loved ones, talk to a trusted friend, or join a support group.

- **Identify your stressors:** Understanding what causes your stress is the first step toward addressing it. Keep a stress diary to monitor your stresses and detect trends.

- **Learn to Say No:** Feel free to establish limits and decline requests that might overwhelm you.

- **Seek Professional Help:** If severe stress interferes with everyday life, try seeing a therapist or counsellor. They may help you develop individualized stress-management methods and improve your overall well-being.

Remember that stress management is a process, not a destination. Be nice to yourself, try various ways, and see what works best for you. By integrating these tools, You may efficiently traverse the storms of stress while cultivating a feeling of serenity and inner peace.

8.3 Importance of Sleep

Sleep. It's more than simply a break; it's an essential symphony in which your body and mind recharge, mend, and prepare for the next day's performance. Just as a well-rested symphony gives a riveting performance, getting enough Sleep helps you to operate at your best, both physically and intellectually. Let's look at why Sleep is so crucial to your general health and well-being.

The first movement is physical restoration.

- **Cellular Renewal:** As you sleep, your body begins to heal itself. Development hormone, which is necessary for cell regeneration and tissue development, is secreted more significantly during Sleep. This not only helps to cure injuries, but it also maintains your skin gleaming and your body working correctly.

- **Muscle Repair and Recovery:** After a long day of physical exertion, Sleep helps your muscles to heal and renew. This is critical for athletes and anybody who regularly exercises.

The second movement involves mental rejuvenation.

Sleep plays an integral part in memory consolidation. During Sleep, your brain absorbs and stores information from the day, converting short-term memories into long-term ones. This helps you learn and remember knowledge more efficiently.

- **Emotional Regulation:** Lack of Sleep may worsen emotional reactions. In contrast, getting enough Sleep helps regulate your emotions, helps you handle stress, and helps you negotiate problems with a more precise and calmer mind.

Third Movement: A Stronger Defense

- **Immune System Boost:** While you sleep, your body creates cytokines, which are proteins that help fight illness and inflammation. This boosts your immune system, making you less prone to disease.

- **Reduced Risk of Chronic Illness:** Chronic sleep deprivation has been associated with an increased risk of chronic illnesses such as cardiovascular disease, diabetes, and obesity. Prioritizing Sleep is an investment in your future health.

The Grand Finale: You Are Well-Rested

Adequate Sleep is essential for a healthy and joyful life. When you're well-rested, you feel:

- **Enhanced Concentration and Focus:** Sleep deprivation may cause fuzzy thinking and difficulties focusing. A good night's Sleep keeps your mind bright and helps you concentrate on things more successfully.

- **Improved Mood and Energy:** Sleep deficiency may cause irritability and sluggishness. Sufficient Sleep fosters a good mood, increases energy levels, and keeps you focused throughout the day.

- **Increased Creativity and Problem-Solving Skills:** When your mind is well-rested, you're more likely to have creative breakthroughs and approach issues from different angles.

Encore: Making Sleep a Priority

Developing proper sleep patterns is critical for receiving a restful night's Sleep. Here are a few tips:

- **Establish a Consistent Sleep Schedule:** Go to bed and wake up simultaneously every day, including weekends. This helps to manage your body's normal sleep-wake cycle.

- **Create a Relaxing Bedtime Routine:** Relax before bedtime with activities such as reading, having a warm bath, or doing mild stretches. Avoid engaging in stimulating activities such as watching television or using technological gadgets.

- Create a Sleep-Conducive Environment. Ensure that your bedroom is dark, quiet, calm, and clutter-free. Invest in a comfy mattress and pillow.

Prioritizing Sleep and implementing good sleep habits into your life helps your body rest and allows it to conduct its nightly symphony of restoration, laying the groundwork for a happier and more satisfying life. So, embrace the power of Sleep and enable it to lead you to a life of ultimate well-being.

Appendix

A1: Glossary of Terms for Hearty Chicken Noodle Soup.

From Hearty Chicken Noodle Soup:

- The broth is a delicious liquid from boiling meat, vegetables, or herbs in water.
- **Sauté:** Quickly sauté food in a tiny quantity of grease over medium heat while stirring constantly.
- Noodles are long, thin pasta strands of wheat and water (or other ingredients).
- Optional: An item or process that might be added or left out according to personal desire.

From baked apples with cinnamon and walnuts:

- The core is the middle section of a fruit or vegetable that includes the seeds or pit.
- Filling is a substance used to pack food before cooking.
- Grated/Zested (citrus peel): A citrus fruit's coarsely crushed or chopped rind is used to enhance its taste.
- Pinch: A minimal quantity, often used for spices or salt.

From Dark Chocolate Avocado Mousse:

- **Double Boiler:** A cooking procedure that involves placing a bowl over simmering water to gradually heat items without burning them.
- Microwaving is the process of heating food using microwave radiation.
- Ripe (avocado): Attained a soft and yielding texture.
- Unsweetened: Omits additional sugar.
- Optional: An item or process that might be added or left out according to personal desire.

Energy balls made with dates, nuts, and seeds:

- Pitted (dates): Having a pit or stone removed.
- Rolled Oats are flattened oat groats that make porridge (oatmeal) or bake.
- **Chopped or diced:** Cut into tiny pieces.
- To chop or ground items, use the food processor's pulse function to switch it on and off momentarily.
- Coating (optional): A coating added to the outside of a food product.

From Exercise and Movement:

- Cardiovascular health refers to the overall health of the heart and blood arteries.
- **Stress reliever:** Something that reduces stress.
- Muscles are the tissues that enable us to move.

- Cognitive function refers to the mental processes that enable people to think, learn, and solve problems.

From Stress Management Techniques:

- Mindfulness is the discipline of paying attention to the present moment without judgment.
- Meditation is a practice aimed at creating a condition of calm and mindfulness.
- Endorphins are hormones generated by the body that reduce pain and improve happiness.
- Negative self-talk includes unhelpful and critical ideas about oneself.
- Gratitude is the emotion of thanks and appreciation.

From The Importance Of Sleep:

- Cellular renewal is replacing older or damaged cells with new ones.
- Cytokines are proteins that help the immune system respond.
- Chronic illnesses are those that develop over an extended period.

A2: Sample Weekly Meal Plans

This example weekly meal plan contains ideas from previous conversations, highlighting culturally inspired cuisine and emphasizing healthy ingredients. Feel free to change the portions and ingredients to suit your tastes and dietary requirements.

Day One (Monday):

- **Breakfast**: Dark Chocolate Avocado Mousse (makes 2-3 serves). A single serving provides a tasty and healthy breakfast. For more texture, top with fresh berries or granola.
- **Lunch**: Leftover Dark Chocolate Avocado Mousse. It may also be consumed as a post-workout snack.
- **Dinner** is Hearty Chicken Noodle Soup (serves 4-6). This soothing soup is ideal for a light meal.

Tuesday (Day 2):

- **Breakfast:** Baked apples with cinnamon and walnuts (serves four). Enjoy a warm, comforting breakfast with a hint of sweetness.
- **Lunch:** Chicken or vegetable salad using leftover chicken from the Hearty Chicken Noodle Soup, diced veggies, and a light vinaigrette dressing.
- **Dinner:** Energy Balls with Dates, Nuts, and Seeds (approximately 15-20 balls). Make a batch of

these energy balls for a nutritious and easy snack or light supper alternative.

Day three (Wednesday):

- **Breakfast:** Oatmeal with chopped nuts and honey. Oatmeal is a traditional morning food that delivers lasting energy.
- **Lunch** is leftover Energy Balls with Dates, Nuts, and Seeds.
- **Dinner:** A vegetarian take on Dark Chocolate Avocado Mousse (optional). If you want a plant-based variation, replace the dark chocolate with a vegan replacement and use nut or seed butter instead.

Day four (Thursday):

- **Breakfast** includes scrambled eggs, chopped veggies, and whole-wheat bread—a protein-rich breakfast to keep you energetic all morning.
- **Lunch:** Salad with grilled chicken or tofu dressed in a mild vinaigrette.
- **Dinner:** Baked apples with cinnamon and walnuts (serves four). Enjoy the warmth and comfort of these baked apples with a delicious supper.

Day five (Friday):

- **Breakfast:** A smoothie with fruits, yoghurt, and spinach. It is a pleasant and healthful way to begin the day.
- **Lunch:** Salad or wrap made with leftover chicken/tofu and veggies.
- **Dinner:** Give yourself a treat! Order takeout from your favourite cuisine or try a new eatery.

Day six (Saturday):

- **Breakfast:** Whole-wheat pancakes or waffles topped with fresh fruit. It is a fun and tasty breakfast option for the weekend.
- **Lunch:** Use leftovers from the week or make a vegetarian Buddha Bowl with roasted veggies, quinoa, and a tahini dressing.
- **Dinner** is Hearty Chicken Noodle Soup (serves 4-6). This warm soup is an excellent way to use leftover chicken from Day 3's salad.

Day seven (Sunday):

- **Breakfast:** French toast baked with whole wheat bread, topped with fresh fruit and maple syrup. It's a delicious brunch choice for a quiet Sunday morning.
- **Lunch:** Light sandwiches prepared with whole wheat bread, lean protein, and veggies.

- **Dinner:** Recreate a meal you especially loved over the week, or try something new!

Snacks:

- Throughout the week, eat nutritious snacks such as fruits, veggies with hummus, nuts and seeds, and yoghurt parfaits.

Drinks:

- Aim for water throughout the day. You may also add unsweetened tea, fruit-infused water, or freshly squeezed juices (in moderation).

This is an example plan; you may modify it depending on your tastes, dietary requirements, and culinary abilities.